MW01028757

'This is perhaps the most th
philosophical basis for nursing practice and nursing c‍‍
date. What is nursing? What sort of people nurses should be? Derek makes this
difficult but important area of nursing inquiry much, much easier. Powerful
and elegant from start to finish, this book should be on the desk of every
nurse.'

— Professor Diana Lee, Chair Professor of Nursing and Director, The
Nethersole School of Nursing, The Chinese University of Hong Kong

'Taking up the conundrum of what constitutes the "good nurse", Derek
Sellman invites us into a lively and intelligent dialogue between science,
morality and applied practice. He guides us underneath our taken-for-
granted understandings of such notions as courage, trustworthiness and open-
mindedness so that we encounter these professional virtues not as fossilised
attributes to be known or possessed, but rather as intricately complex,
delicately situated, and constantly evolving expressions of human practices
within the conditions that shape them. Teasing apart the ideals these virtues
represent, he challenges our usual approaches to thinking about the nature
of nursing, encouraging us to reframe the manner in which we educate those
who seek to learn the mysteries of its practice.'

— Professor Sally Thorne, University of British Columbia
School of Nursing, Vancouver, Canada

'Derek Sellman's text is both a timely and highly absorbing journey deep into
the heart of nursing. It reveals a timeless and essential set of key virtues that
should be a major part of the moral compass of every nurse. Consequently, it
should be read by all nurses – and most certainly by all nurse educators – who
are interested in maintaining and promoting the vital moral characteristics of
nursing now and in the future.'

— Dr Martin Woods, Senior Lecturer, School of Health and
Social Services, Massey University, New Zealand

'Nursing, according to Derek Sellman, is a MacIntyrian practice which
can only flourish when it is not prevented from pursuing the completion
of independent ideas. In *What Makes a Good Nurse*, being vulnerable,
trustworthy and open-minded are central virtues studied critically to offer
future perspectives. Situated in the realities of the nursing profession today,
Sellman draws on his rich experiences as a teacher of nursing and his deep
reflections as a philosopher. This is what makes the book so authentic and
easy to stroll through the realms of philosophy. Readers will certainly feel
encouraged to engage in a fruitful conversation on moral understandings of
contemporary professional nursing.'

— Dr Helen Kohlen, Sociologist, Junior Professor of Care Policy and
Ethics, Faculty of Nursing, University of Vallendar, Germany

Emerging Values in Health Care
The Challenge for Professionals
Edited by Stephen Pattison, Ben Hannigan, Roisin Pill and Huw Thomas
ISBN 978 1 84310 947 1

Making Sense of Spirituality in Nursing and Health Care Practice
An Interactive Approach
2nd edition
Wilfred McSherry
Foreword by Keith Cash
ISBN 978 1 84310 365 3

Medicine of the Person
Faith, Science and Values in Health Care Provision
Edited by John Cox, Alastair V. Campbell and Bill K. W. M. Fulford
Foreword by Julia Neuberger
ISBN 978 1 84310 397 4

Talking About Spirituality in Health Care Practice
A Resource for the Multi-Professional Health Care Team
Gillian White
ISBN 978 1 84310 305 9

Spirituality, Ethics and Care
Simon Robinson
ISBN 978 1 84310 498 8

Working Relationships
Spirituality in Human Service and Organisational Life
Neil Pembroke
ISBN 978 1 84310 252 6

What Makes a Good Nurse

Why the Virtues are Important for Nurses

Derek Sellman

Foreword by Alan Cribb

Jessica Kingsley *Publishers*
London and Philadelphia

Please see page 14 for a full list of permissions granted.

First published in 2011
by Jessica Kingsley Publishers
116 Pentonville Road
London N1 9JB, UK
and
400 Market Street, Suite 400
Philadelphia, PA 19106, USA

www.jkp.com

Copyright © Derek Sellman 2011
Foreword copyright © Alan Cribb 2011

Library of Congress Cataloging in Publication Data
Sellman, Derek.
What makes a good nurse : why the virtues are important for nurses / Derek
Sellman ; foreword by Alan Cribb.
p. ; cm.
Includes bibliographical references and index.
ISBN 978-1-84310-932-7 (alk. paper)
1. Nursing--Philosophy. 2. Values. I. Title.
[DNLM: 1. Nurse's Role. 2. Ethics, Nursing. WY 87]
RT42.S45 2011
610.73--dc22
2010045495

British Library Cataloguing in Publication Data
A CIP catalogue record for this book is available from the British Library

ISBN 978 1 84310 932 7

Printed and bound in Great Britain

*To Louise, Tom, Joe and Imogen for
your patience and support*

In memory of Paul Wainwright 1948–2010

Contents

Foreword

Those of us who are lucky enough to have friends who are nurses know that, in broad terms, it is the character qualities that we admire in them that go towards making them good nurses. Similarly, those of us who are lucky enough to have been taken care of and treated by nurses know that the admirable character qualities (or 'virtues') of these nurses are absolutely central to what makes them good nurses – it is about 'who they are' and not just 'what they do'. Yet, as Derek Sellman shows in this book, and helps us understand in the pages that follow, there is a serious 'disconnect' between these familiar personal judgements and so much of the educational, managerial and even professional language of nursing. One key symbol of this disconnect is the fact that, although in the UK (at least) a 'declaration of good character' signed by an assessor is required before someone can be registered as a nurse, comparatively little thought goes into such a signature (and into consideration of what such a declaration means) and nearly all of the substantial thought and care that rightly goes into the education and assessment of prospective nurses is invested elsewhere.

This disconnect is a familiar and pervasive one. When we describe the people we admire and care about in our personal lives many of us find it natural to celebrate their character; but when we have to 'appraise' our colleagues at work we are often forced into talking in a strange and impoverished language. In the former instance we might comfortably talk about a friend's remarkable compassion, courage and integrity but in the latter instance we can sometimes be required to talk in terms of our colleagues' 'competences' and 'transferable skills' and perhaps their contribution to 'key performance indicators'. This impoverishment of language is a surface sign of a serious underlying malaise. This book is an important one because it helps us to recognise, understand and respond constructively to this malaise.

The gap between what people know matters (at a personal level) and what they feel able to talk about (in a professional context) arises in part because they are often unsure how to talk about virtues, or because they find such talk uncomfortable or embarrassing, or even because they feel it is actually wrong – old-fashioned, elitist, 'judgemental'. Sellman's careful analysis shows us how mistaken and potentially damaging these feelings and perceptions are. He explains and defends the unequivocal importance of professional virtues in nursing, and offers us insights not only into the nature of the virtues but into their philosophical foundations and their ethical and practical centrality.

Sellman's call for a renewed emphasis on character and on 'practical wisdom' involves a process of recovery. It is about recovering and renewing a language capable of making fundamental and essential discriminations about what it is we do, and ought to aim to be doing, in our work and lives. But it is not primarily a process of linguistic recovery – it is about wiser ways of seeing the world and of being in the world, about different possible futures within nursing and health care and, for that matter, within our societies too.

Professor Alan Cribb
Centre for Public Policy Research
King's College London
February 2011

Acknowledgements

There are so many individuals to whom I am indebted for the production of this book that it would be impossible to name them all. This is partly because, as I note in my preface, the book is the result of many conversations held at many different locations with many different people over many years. Almost all of these conversations remain transient and unrecorded but they have all in their way shaped my thinking and writing. Despite the wealth of conversations that underpin this book there are some that stand out as significant and it is for these that I try to name those individuals who have been instrumental in what appears here, although it is important to note that I take sole responsibility for any errors that appear in the text.

In this regard I would like to thank in particular Paul Wainwright whose friendship and encouragement over many years was invaluable – Paul also developed an account of nursing as a practice, in the sense that the philosopher Alasdair MacIntyre uses that term, in his PhD and I am grateful for his generosity and critical engagement on this topic. I thank Graham Haydon who was instrumental in setting me off in this direction and Patricia White who so gracefully supervised my PhD. Thanks are owed to those whose conversations have inspired me in this work and, mindful of the danger of neglecting those who deserve a mention (and apologies in advance to anyone who falls into that category), I thank, in no particular order: Ann Gallagher, Steven Edwards, John Drummond, John Paley, Stephen Pattison, Trevor Hussey, John White, Terrance McLaughlin, Janet Holt, Paul Snelling, Martin Lipscomb, Mark Risjord, Peter Allmark and Alan Cribb for their sometimes inspiring insights and conversations.

I would also like to thank Jessica Kingsley for encouraging me to put these ideas together in a single volume and I am grateful to her for providing this opportunity to publish. I am also grateful to those publishers who have allowed me to draw extensively from my own previously published work in the compilation of this book. Thus I am grateful for the permissions given as follows:

I thank Wiley-Blackwell for permission to reproduce and amend for the purposes of completing this book the following articles: D. Sellman (2000) 'Alasdair MacIntyre and the professional practice of nursing.' *Nursing Philosophy 1*, 1, 26–33; D. Sellman (2003) 'Open-mindedness: a virtue for professional practice.' *Nursing Philosophy 4*, 1, 17–24; D. Sellman (2005) 'Towards an understanding of nursing as a response to human vulnerability.' *Nursing Philosophy 6*, 1, 2–10; D. Sellman (2007) 'Trusting patients, trusting nurses.' *Nursing Philosophy 8*, 1, 28–36; and D. Sellman (2009) 'Vulnerability and nursing: a reply to Havi Carel.' *Nursing Philosophy 10*, 3, 220–222.

I also thank SAGE Publications for permission to republish the whole or any part of the article that first appeared as 'The importance of being trustworthy'. The final definitive version of this paper has been published in *Nursing Ethics 13*, 2 (2006) by SAGE Publications Ltd. All rights reserved ©, available at http://nej.sagepub.com/content/13/2/105.

Similarly, I would like to thank Troubador Publishing for permission to reproduce here my work published originally as D. Sellman (2008) 'Teaching Ethics to Nurses in Higher Education: Just Another Subject or an Exercise in Moral Education?' In S. Robinson and J. Strain (eds) *Ethics for Working and Living*. Leicester: Troubador Publishing, pp.108–120.

Preface

This book represents the written culmination of a conversation that started many years ago when I was asked by a ward-based mentor how she should go about undertaking the practice assessment of a student who was technically proficient but had an uncertain set of attitudes; attitudes that this particular mentor thought inappropriate for nursing. The guidance I was able to offer this mentor in her assessment of that particular student was predicated on the criteria by which student assessment in practice was measured in that institution at that time. Even as the mentor assessed (and passed) the student it was clear to both the mentor and myself that there was something unsatisfactory about a process in which student success could occur, apparently, in the absence of any concerns with the character of a student. The conversation has since taken many turns and has included episodes that are seemingly unrelated as well as those that are obviously related to this concern. I have occupied a variety of roles in the academy during this time and the students, colleagues, managers, educators, scholars and others with whom I have conversed have all in their way contributed to the writing that I present here in this book.

Some parts of the conversation in this book will be recognisable to those readers who are familiar with my work for this book does indeed draw from and extend those earlier conversational snippets that have already appeared in print. One of the features of this book is that it puts together some of these previously published ideas into an overall framework that makes sense to me and, I hope, to the reader.

I would like to be able to say that the publication of the book represents the end of this particular conversation. But I know better than to make a claim of this sort for even as I write this preface, and with the manuscript complete and ready to be sent to the publisher, I am aware of several areas of the conversation that would benefit from further exploration, justification, clarification, discussion, argumentation and/ or expansion. I also know that the project has already taken many years to get to this stage and despite recognising that one danger of publication is the possibility of the fossilisation of ideas, it just feels about the right sort of time to unleash the conversation in its current form. That the conversation will continue I have no doubt, and I hope that I will be able to contribute further at some future time. I hope, too, that others will want to further this conversation and, while I hesitate to commit to another book-size argument, I can even now sense that there are several directions in which this conversation might proceed and any one of these routes might provide fertile ground for a sequel (so to speak). However, right now (with the recent memory of the all-consuming nature of finishing a manuscript at the forefront of my thinking), starting over with the whole process of writing another book does not seem a particularly sensible thing to do. However, even without a book-sized project in mind the conversation will continue and I know that at some point my fingers will begin to work the keyboard once more to record some of the thoughts that come with the continuing conversation. I hope too that the reader will be encouraged to similarly engage with and develop the conversation.

Derek Sellman
Edmonton, Alberta
October 2010

Introduction

Assuming that most people have an idea of the type of work nurses do, it is not unreasonable to suppose they would also be inclined to anticipate nurses ought to be caring, compassionate, trustworthy and so on as they go about their daily work. This is to say that most people expect a nurse not only to have the appropriate set of task skills for nursing but also to have a particular set of characteristics; that is, character traits consistent with caring for others. This suggests that people assume caring to be a central feature of nursing practice; a view that, generally speaking, corresponds with the views held by nurses themselves. Indeed the idea of an uncaring nurse is particularly unappealing and is as likely to draw censure as the idea of an unskilled nurse.

It is the general experience (and expectation) of admission tutors for nursing programmes that candidates express a desire to be of help to others as a primary reason for wishing to become a nurse. Given both the history of altruistic motivation for practice and the enduring idea of caring as a central feature of nursing it might be supposed that the philosophical basis for nursing practice and nursing education had long been satisfactorily worked out; after all everybody seems to think they know just what it is that nurses do and what sort of people nurses should be. Unfortunately, ongoing debates that reflect fundamental disagreements about the nature of nursing as well as about the proper aims of nursing practice demonstrate that the philosophical basis of nursing is far from uncontentious. And this has inevitable implications for both the general and moral education of nurses.

This book is offered as a contribution to the philosophical basis for nursing practice and nursing education. I will argue that nursing is an inherently moral practice and that this places moral obligations on individual nurses to cultivate the sorts of dispositions necessary to ensure nursing actions enable rather than diminish human flourishing. Expressed in this way these sentiments might seem merely to reflect long cherished ideals of nursing, yet, as will be seen, the application of these ideals both in the practice and in the education of nurses is far from straightforward. Among the features of this book that impact directly on the practice and education of nurses, five are of particular interest.

First, I note the unsatisfactory way in which the idea of the vulnerability of recipients of nursing practice is expressed. This leads towards a preliminary analysis of the nature of human vulnerability and from this I develop the notion of the *more-than-ordinarily* vulnerable person. This is to say that we are all vulnerable but there is an additional vulnerability that comes with being a patient and means that patients are, by definition, *more-than-ordinarily* vulnerable. And this is one reason why it is important for nurses to cultivate what might be termed 'protective' virtues in pursuit of the flourishing of patients.

Second, the idea that nurses should be trustworthy seems to be accepted as a generally unproblematic notion. However, being trustworthy as a nurse is complicated because of the diverse range of expectations from patients, relatives, colleagues, managers, peers, regulatory and professional bodies, and the institutions within which nursing practice takes place. Nurses are often faced with competing demands and sometimes the same action will be perceived as trustworthy from the perspective of one party but as untrustworthy from the perspective of another party. This means being trustworthy as a nurse requires the use of professional judgement and discretion in the complex practical situations in which nurses find themselves. In Aristotelian terms such professional judgement approximates *phronesis* (practical wisdom).

Third, and drawing from Terence McLaughlin's idea of *pedagogic phronesis* (McLauglin 2003a), I suggest that it makes sense to describe the *phronesis* necessary for professional practice as *professional phronesis*. In so doing I am casting what nursing's regulatory bodies (including the UK Nursing and Midwifery Council (NMC)) refer to as professional judgement (the centrepiece of professional accountability) as *professional phronesis* (Sellman 2009). If I am right about this then one of the aims of nursing education is that it should prepare students to learn how to become the *professional phronimos* (the professionally wise person) (Sellman 2009). In the Aristotelian sense *phronesis* is a centrally important virtue and any curriculum that seeks to develop virtue in students must take seriously the idea of a moral education fundamentally associated with the cultivation of virtue.

Fourth, and following on from the above, I advance the idea of the necessity of a moral education for nurses. This idea of the moral education of nurses might seem odd for (at least) two related reasons. First, students of nursing are adults and it is more usual to find children, rather than adults, the focus of discussions about moral education. Second, in the majority of developed countries at least, nursing education is formally located within institutions of higher education and the general assumption is that higher education involves learning and teaching in relation to particular and discrete subject areas rather than a concern with the character of the student. Nevertheless, regulatory bodies for nursing do indicate implicitly, if not explicitly, the need for those admitted to professional registers of nurses to be of good character (see, for example, NMC 2008a; CARNA 2010).

Fifth, I consider what it means for a nurse to be of good character. Nursing's regulatory bodies do have an interest in the character of registered nurses and this is made more explicit in some regions than in others. In the UK the NMC requires that those responsible for pre-registration nursing education in the UK sign a declaration of good health and *good character* before a student who has otherwise successfully completed the preparatory course is allowed to register as a nurse (NMC 2008a). In the province of Alberta in Canada, the College and Association of Registered Nurses of Alberta (CARNA) requires registrants to confirm their good character and reputation at annual renewal of license to practice (CARNA 2010). If nurses are required to be of good character it is reasonable to expect that regulatory bodies spell out exactly what is meant by this, if only so that those charged with preparatory nursing education can design curricula appropriately and know how it is that they are supposed to assess the good character of aspiring and existing registered nurses. As it stands, nursing's regulatory bodies seem to understand good character as the absence of criminal or unprofessional behaviour; neither is it clear how and when nurse educators are to assess students' characters. In arguing the case for a virtue ethics conception of the moral education of nurses this book makes a contribution to exploring the idea of a good character suitable for nursing practice and therefore suitable as a model by which nurse educators might aim to cultivate the appropriate sorts of caring virtues in students of nursing.

These five themes are threaded throughout this book as I develop the idea of nursing as a practice in the sense that Alasdair MacIntyre (1985) uses that term. A number of authors have argued that teaching is a practice in this sense (see, for example, Dunne 2003) and in Chapter 3 I argue that there is benefit to be gained in understanding nursing as a MacIntyrean practice; a practice, moreover, that is a social, moral and professional practice. In this respect teaching and nursing (along with a number of other occupational groups) share some common moral grounding for their practice. As such, much that will be said in this book will be applicable to both teaching and nursing (as well as to other similar types of occupations) although it should be recognised from the outset that differences between these individual practices do exist. Because the main focus of this book is the practice of nursing, considerations of teaching as a practice are limited to those discussions that contribute to development of moral practitioners of nursing.

Nursing, like teaching, contends with a number of internal and external pressures, some of which have the potential to undermine basic assumptions about the practice itself. External pressures come thick and fast in terms of policy directives, targets, the need to demonstrate value for money and so on. Internal pressures arise in large measure from a seeming inability of nursing to define itself and, in particular, from the positioning of some practitioners and scholars who pursue an ideal of nursing science as a corollary to medical science. It is one of my contentions that this concentration of effort on the development of a discrete nursing science is misguided and, moreover, threatens conceptions of nursing as a response to human vulnerability. It is true that science has much to offer nursing but to consider nursing as solely a science, or as merely a set of technical tasks to be accomplished, is to misunderstand the nature of nursing. Nursing is not, and can never be, merely a set of prescribed skills precisely because the human condition makes it unlikely that any interaction with a patient will ever be merely a matter of routine. In addition to being professional, interactions between nurses and patients are inevitably (inter)personal and as such there is a need to resist those pressures that might incline nurses to view patients as just so many widgets to be processed through a service or as customers of a store. While store workers may engage in 'customer care', such care is more likely to originate from instrumental and commercial interests rather than from any primary concern for the best interests of the customer. Hence, while there are some moral constraints in any form of service, there are additional moral expectations of nurses and other health care professionals as compared to those of other service industry workers. In this book I attempt to identify what it is that places nursing in the category of occupations in which practitioners are expected to uphold particular (and generally higher than everyday) moral standards.

Neglect of its moral content does a disservice to nursing as an occupation, to individual nurses, and to individual patients. Consequently, I place moral considerations, and in particular matters of character, at the core of nursing practice and nursing education. In so doing questions about the nature and purpose(s) of nursing as well as questions about what makes a good nurse inevitably arise. In addressing these questions it will become clear that on the account offered in this book, a good nurse is one who exhibits certain sorts of virtues and, for reasons that will be made explicit, I have adopted the term *professional virtue* to describe these virtues (Sellman 2000). No attempt is made in this book to list every professional virtue that might be thought necessary for the practice of nursing, rather a number of core professional virtues are identified and two are discussed in detail.

A note on nomenclature

It should be noted at the outset that the term 'patient' is not universally accepted as an appropriate word to describe individuals in receipt of nursing care. Some nurses prefer the term client on the grounds that it implies a less passive relationship on the part of the person in receipt of health care. Some take client to describe a partnership *between* a practitioner and a client rather than a form of paternalism where actions are undertaken *by* a professional *on* rather than *with* a patient. Generally speaking in the UK nurses working with adults who have some physical illness tend to use the term 'patient', nurses working in the area of mental health tend to talk about 'clients', nurses working with people with learning difficulties often consider their client group as 'service users', and children's nurses tend to consider their client group as children within a family unit.

The phrase 'patient and/or client' or 'patient/client' is sometimes used in the literature but it is my view that this tends to add an awkwardness and, in some cases, an unnecessary complexity to ideas under discussion. The debate on whether or not persons in receipt of health care are best described as patients, clients, service users or by some other designation arises, at least in part, because of the breadth of health and nursing care provision. While the term 'patient' would be generally accepted as appropriate to use for a person admitted to a general hospital for surgery, the term 'client' might better describe the person admitted as an emergency to a mental health facility. For the sake of simplicity and clarity the terms 'patient', 'client', 'service user' and 'recipient of care' will be used throughout this book as synonymous and interchangeable to denote any individual who is in receipt of nursing practice.

A note on definitional difficulties for nursing

Nursing is a demanding activity. In the UK there are over 600,000 registered nurses providing nursing care 24 hours a day, seven days a week, 52 weeks a year. It might be thought that with so many individuals occupied in the activity there would exist a fairly clear idea about the nature of nursing. However, the debate about terminology crystallises some of the tensions about how nursing is understood and the tendency to consider nurses as a homogeneous group is to mistake the scope of nursing practice. Nursing covers such a wide variety of activities that it is difficult to encapsulate what nurses do in any simple statement. While in the UK there are four distinct fields of nursing (adult nursing; children's nursing; learning disabilities nursing; and mental health nursing) these areas of practice, together with elements of maternal care in some countries, are universally included in what nurses do. However, even this categorisation does not sufficiently identify the full range or focus of activity undertaken by nurses, for there is a bewildering array of roles within and between each client group area (for example, community nurses, hospital nurses, nurse administrators, practice nurses, consultant nurses, research nurses, clinical nurse specialists, nurse educators, occupational health nurses and so on). This breadth of activity represents both a spectrum of nursing services and a range of institutions in which nursing takes place. Thus while many nurses will take it as read that they are caring for patients in a predominately medical environment, many others will consider that medicine has little to do with the nursing care required by, for example, someone whose reason for being in receipt of nursing care is either non-medical (for example, someone with learning disabilities) or incurable (in any medical sense). The role of a nurse in caring for persons so described might include providing assistance in living outside of an institution or help in maximising potential for self-determination. It should be evident from this brief discussion that there is no simple definition of either what it means to be a nurse or of what is understood by the term 'nursing' and more detailed consideration is given to this in Chapter 3. For now it is sufficient to recognise the complexity of nursing and to suggest that one thing that nurses have in common is a concern for the well-being of persons in receipt of their practice.

A note on nursing codes

Since publication of the first International Council of Nurses (ICN) Code of Ethics in 1953 many countries have developed their own nursing code. These codes go by various names (for example, codes of professional practice, codes of ethics and so on) and are designed perhaps with slightly different primary purposes (for example, regulatory, disciplinary and so on). Nevertheless, these codes share not only a common antecedent in the ICN Code but also a common grounding in the values that are said to be fundamental to conceptions of nursing. Like other professional codes, nursing codes are subject to revision over time and this trend is set to continue as codes are reviewed in response to societal and other changes. Hence, amendments to nursing codes tend to be changes in emphasis and language rather than changes to core nursing values. Readers should therefore anticipate that quotes used in this book that originate from nursing codes are used primarily for illustrative purposes. This is to say that while current at the time of writing, quotes used from individual nursing codes may well be out of date at the time of reading. However, it is my view that regardless of the actual words used, the fundamental values of nursing can be found in all nursing codes, regardless of time and place. In other words, while the choice of quotes from nursing codes used in this book (and because of my background I draw primarily from the UK code) may seem to be out of date, readers should anticipate that the same sentiments can be found, albeit in different words, in their own current nursing code.

Structure and content of the book

Chapter 1 introduces the idea that, contrary to expectation, the teaching of ethics to students of nursing does not necessarily lead to the development of ethical practitioners. The reasons for this are explored and it is argued that this failure of ethics to develop the appropriate virtues requires an explicit moral education for nurses. An outline of, and some preliminary justification for, the general Aristotelian approach adopted is offered together with a response to a particularly strong challenge to the whole idea of a virtue ethics. Chapter 2 proceeds with a discussion of human vulnerability in general and in relation to the position of those who are or who become the recipients of nursing practise in particular. I argue that patients are *more-than-ordinarily* vulnerable and that being *more-than-ordinarily* vulnerable compromises possibilities for human flourishing in ways that being ordinarily vulnerable does not. From this I argue that one legitimate aim of nursing is to encourage human flourishing; in other words, this is to say that nursing can be understood, at least in part, as a response to particular aspects of human vulnerability. And because of this it is helpful for nurses to cultivate and exhibit certain sorts of professional virtues.

Chapter 3 begins with an argument against the idea that nursing is a science and against the idea that the development of some kind of a pure nursing science is either possible or desirable. I argue that nursing is better served by being understood as a practice in the technical sense in which Alastair MacIntyre (1985) employs that term to denote particular forms of human activity in which the virtues may flourish. I then go on to consider MacIntyre's account of human flourishing together with some implications for nursing practice. The chapter concludes with a brief overview of the place of MacIntyre's core virtues of courage, truthfulness and justice in the practice of nursing. Chapter 4 offers an account of the nature of trust and trustworthiness and the place of both in the practice of nursing. I argue that while there are substantial difficulties with the idea of trustworthiness as a virtue as such, it can, nevertheless, be considered as a professional virtue at least in the terms is which I define professional virtue. I argue that despite a general acceptance of the need for nurses (and other health care practitioners) to be trustworthy, what is meant by trustworthiness in professional life is poorly articulated. I argue that professional trustworthiness is essential to the moral practice of nursing and as such is a core professional virtue.

Chapter 5 develops the argument that in addition to trustworthiness, open-mindedness is another essential, although often neglected, professional virtue. I argue that many of the problems that beset nursing practice (and nursing education) result from failures of open-mindedness. Failures of open-mindedness are of two kinds: 1) those failures that result from a general attitude of closed- or narrow-mindedness, and 2) those failures that result from a tendency to credulousness. Some of the conceptual and practical difficulties in aiming for open-mindedness, and the implications for the ethical practice of nursing are discussed. Chapter 6 attempts to consider what sort of approach to the education of nurses is most likely to encourage the development of those professional virtues appropriate for nursing. Inevitably this discussion is constrained by the difficulties of providing suitable evidence for the claims made but this should not be considered as a fatal obstacle to the discussion. If it is true that nurses must be more than mere technicians or mere deliverers of packages of care then the debate about how best to educate for moral practice is of the utmost importance and cannot wait until compelling evidence for change is available. The ways in which nursing knowledge, nursing education and nursing practice are conceptualised, organised and delivered will inevitably affect the ways in which students and practitioners of nursing are encouraged or discouraged in the cultivation of virtues and/or vices. And because this is of such importance for the well-being of patients it is essential that the debate about the moral education of nurses is not neglected.

The conclusion briefly summarises how the arguments of this book contribute to and have a practical bearing on nursing practice, nursing education and nursing codes.

1 Professional Nursing

Given that, at least in general terms, existing arrangements for nurse education are well established it might be thought that the issue of character development for nurses is unproblematic. If this were true then an investigation into aspects of the moral education of nurses would be unnecessary and unproductive. However, as I shall argue, current arrangements for the education of nurses do little to encourage the development of those character traits (care, compassion, trustworthiness and so on) that it is assumed nurses will exhibit. Indeed, it might be reasonably anticipated that a programme of study designed to lead to qualification as a nurse would place emphasis on character development as well as on skill acquisition and it might then come as a surprise to find so little time devoted to notions of, for example, care, compassion and trustworthiness in the nursing curricula. There is a professional aspiration for character development that can be found among the various nursing codes found in the developed world and within the supporting documents that go along with these codes, made explicit by the requirement for those who wish to become registered nurses to be of good character as a condition of entry to nursing registers. It is not, then, that the character of a nurse is ignored, rather it is that whatever being of good character requires remains poorly articulated.

However, it would be to overstate the case to say that issues of morally acceptable behaviour are neglected in nursing curricula for one feature of programmes of preparation for nursing is a requirement for the inclusion of professional ethics. We might then be reassured that the teaching of ethics to nurses ensures that nurses learn to become ethical practitioners but this, of course, depends on how the teaching of ethics is undertaken, and on how far it is reasonable to imagine that the teaching of ethics leads to the development of ethical practitioners.

The teaching of ethics to nurses

Ethics is part of nursing curricula. However, there is anecdotal evidence to suggest that students of nursing (and nurses generally) accept a hierarchy of subjects with the natural sciences at the pinnacle providing the sources of 'hard evidence' for 'real knowledge' and other subjects areas somehow 'softer' and of less importance. In nursing education generally, ethics and professional issues are often perceived as part of that 'softer' set of subjects and many students seem to consider these subjects as optional. But there is nothing soft about ethical and professional matters; indeed such matters go to the heart of the purposes of nursing. The nature of nursing work brings human vulnerability into sharp relief and with it a whole range of questions about which nursing actions best meet the needs of patients; questions that are among the most difficult to answer precisely because they deal with essential problems of human frailty. As a consequence ethical and professional issues remain of central concern to the enterprise of nursing. It follows then that there needs to be some form of ethics content in programmes of study leading to professional nurse registration, and this is often taken to mean that the teaching of ethics to nurses should be a subject in its own right. But before exploring what this means for nurse education, a brief historical detour might provide some useful contextual information.

The tradition of ethics in nursing during most of the twentieth century owes much to Florence Nightingale, although as I have argued elsewhere (Sellman 1997) much of that which is generally regarded as reactionary in Nightingale stems from some rather narrow interpretations and over-simplified sound bites. Nevertheless, the generally accepted wisdom is that Nightingale's legacy left ethics for nurses in a sorry state and even as far into the twentieth century as the early 1970s material was published under the heading of ethics for nurses that might be better and more accurately described as etiquette for nurses. The following extract is of a not uncommon tenor:

> Ward routine has a certain pattern to encourage respect for the doctor: he is always accompanied by the sister, the ward is quiet, he is never contradicted; and by various means he is shown to be a person of pre-eminent skill and wisdom. (Wray 1962, p.22)

Thus, in the UK at least, the teaching of ethics as anything other than etiquette to nurses is of relatively recent origin. The emergence of the current sense of ethics and professional issues as necessary for the professional practice of nursing in the UK can be located within the debates about accountability of the late 1970s and early 1980s which preceded the introduction of the first UK code of conduct for nurses from the United Kingdom Central Council for Nurses, Midwifery and Health Visiting (UKCC) (UKCC 1983). This explicit requirement for the inclusion of ethics in the pre-registration nursing curricula was formalised as part of the 'Project 2000' re-imagining of nursing education from the late 1980s (UKCC 1986) and introduced at a time when nurse education was beginning the move from hospital-based schools of nursing towards incorporation into higher education. This required a cultural change as nurse teachers who had previously been generalists (that is, taught whatever needed teaching) found themselves required to teach to a specialism. Consequently, many nurse teachers were forced to adopt or develop particular subject expertise in order to teach, for example, anatomy and physiology, sociology, psychology, ethics and so on to nurses. That many nurse teachers were ill prepared as subject specialist teachers in ethics is witnessed by the development of courses aimed at just such nurse teachers.[1] This lack of a tradition of formal ethics teaching in nursing education may help to account for the continuing debates about the purpose(s) of teaching ethics to nurses (see, for example, Holt and Long 1999; NMC 2004; Scott 1995; Sellman 1996; Woods 2005; Woogara 2005).

Nevertheless, the teaching of ethics to nurses tends to take the form of the necessary learning of a subject matter that can be applied to practice situations in just the same way as, for example, the learning of physiology or psychology. As a result there is a tendency to teach ethics theory in the form of, for example, principles, rights theory, deontology or utilitarianism and this is certainly how health care ethics is presented in many popular ethics textbooks (see, for example, Beauchamp and Childress 2008; Edwards 2009; Gillon 1985; Thompson, Melia and Boyd 2000). And while some more than others of these texts offer discussion of ethical matters they generally do so from a position that might be described as attempts to work out what to do when certain types of situations arise. Indeed, some (see, for example, Seedhouse 2009) provide models for ethical decision-making. This reflects an emphasis of the 'application of theory' approach to professional education and assumes that the intellectualisation of matters ethical will lead to reasoned moral action. While it is indeed appropriate to rehearse and debate ethical positions on, for example, whether or not one should lie to patients in order to assist students to engage with a variety of theoretical perspectives, it is not clear that the teaching of ethics in this modern sense as an academic subject can lead to reasoned moral action. The teaching of ethics as a discrete subject (sometimes conceived as the teaching of professional issues or as teaching for accountability) assumes that students who understand what it means to be an accountable professional will behave in ways that reflect behaviour born of an internalisation of the NMC code.[2] But the idea that teaching the knowledge base of ethics will result in more ethically-oriented persons is unsustainable for, as Baier (1985) reminds us, such teaching is as likely to encourage scepticism as morality. In nursing there is evidence of a similar failure to connect teaching and learning of ethics with moral behaviour. As Scott puts it:

> some nurse theorists have been misled in that they have confused the actual process of moral development with theories *about* this process. This results in the claim that, if Kohlberg's theory of moral development is used as a framework in nursing education, it will lead to high levels of moral action by student nurses and thus, as students qualify, to high quality moral behaviour among practitioners. (Scott 1995, p.282; original emphasis)

Thus one danger of the teaching of ethics as a discrete subject area is that it can have the effect of intellectualising issues of moral consequence. The temptation to teach ethics in ways that relate to ethical issues generated by the rise of science and the accompanying technological advances also presents a danger. This approach might be described as a 'big issues' approach to ethics and features large in what has come to be known as medical or bioethics. While interesting in themselves and for society generally, the big issues of ethics are of less direct relevance to the everyday practice of the majority of health care professionals than might be imagined. As such, teaching that emphasises these types of ethical problems (issues related to biogenetics, abortion, euthanasia and so on) tends to portray ethics as an abstract subject largely divorced from the everyday practice of nurses. And because these approaches tend to follow the purported scientific view that emotion should give way to reason, the teaching of ethics undertaken from these perspectives cannot provide a proper foundation for moral education. Hence while the teaching of ethics has much to contribute towards nursing students' understanding of professional and ethical obligations it does not, of itself, provide sufficient grounding for the development of the kind of character traits that are considered appropriate or even necessary for nurse practitioners. In other words, teaching ethics (in the sense of a discrete academic subject) cannot function as or replace a moral education designed to cultivate those very particular virtues necessary for the ethical practice of nursing.

Moral guidance

While the teaching of ethics to nurses may contribute to nursing students' knowledge and understanding of morality, what I have termed the 'application of theory' approaches thus far discussed do not and cannot constitute moral education as here conceived. Thus it seems that something more that the mere teaching of ethics is a necessary component of nursing education if the expectation that nurses exhibit certain sorts of caring dispositions can be met. In other words, in addition to the teaching of ethics there is a requirement for some form of moral guidance or moral education. However, Holt and Long reject the idea of moral guidance as they argue that it is precisely the teaching of ethics as a subject just like any other subject that is necessary if nursing students are to be able to make ethical judgements 'supported by good reasons for accepting a belief if such judgements are to be considered more than just simple opinions' (Holt and Long 1999, p.247). Further they argue for training in philosophical method of 'how to critically evaluate the beliefs and arguments advanced on ethical issues' (p.247) and this is, of course, necessary if nurses are to be able to spot fallacious arguments supporting questionable practices. Holt and Long's discussion is partly an attack on 'armchair' ethicist approaches to the teaching of ethics where abstract ethical theory is used to proclaim judgements from afar in ways that students of nursing will find obscure and divorced from their clinical experiences; and Holt and Long are quite right to emphasise the need to locate ethical discussion in the framework of clinical practice if such discussion is to be meaningful to nursing students. But they go on to differentiate between on the one hand the teaching of ethics as a legitimate activity and on the other an inappropriate and unhelpful tendency of nurse educators to give moral guidance. They do not clarify exactly what they mean by 'moral guidance' but it can inferred from their argument that they use the term to indicate teaching that gives prominence to 'imposing…lists of acceptable behaviour' (p.249): an approach that might be likened to moral training rather than moral education. And if this is what they mean then they are correct in saying that mere moral guidance is unhelpful in the education of nurses because it is inconsistent with the educational aim of enabling nurses to engage in independent practical reasoning in order to determine what should be done to whom in difficult clinical situations.

Holt and Long claim that moral guidance may be an acceptable function of teachers of primary school children because children of such age have not sufficiently developed the cognitive capacities necessary for moral reasoning. This view seems to be underpinned by a Kohlbergian approach to moral education, which 'character educators accuse…of concentrating exclusively on moral process to the neglect of moral content' (Noddings and Slote 2003, p.351). Holt and Long's argument also appears be overly paternalistic and fails to recognise that the development of young children's critical moral capacities requires more than mere guidance from authority adult figures. At the very least it needs a nurturing environment where 'good' reasons for morally acceptable behaviour can be explored and discussed in terms with which the children can engage. Hugh Sockett (1993, pp.1–3) provides a telling illustration of the very moral reasoning of which Holt and Long seem to think young children are incapable. Sockett describes how, in a few brief, unscheduled, moments, a teacher engages a group of 30 five-year-old school children in discussion about acceptable moral behaviour in relation to a particular issue unrelated to the ongoing class work. The teacher could have merely told the children that such and such was out of bounds for the day but instead she helped the children to work out for themselves why it was necessary not to go near a particular part of the classroom for the rest of that day. This is no mere 'moral guidance' in the sense in which Holt and Long have used that term; neither did the teacher think of it as teaching in ethics. But it was a form of moral education that enabled those five-year-old children to link together reason and action in the pursuit of individual and common good.

Holt and Long state: 'moral guidance as a strategy is unacceptable, and that a basic introduction to philosophical methods is the key to effective learning of the skills required for autonomous analysis and decision making.' (Holt and Long 1999, p.246). They are, of course, quite right to note that in developing skills of philosophical method students will be able to engage in autonomous decision-making but the binary contrast is inaccurate and incomplete. Holt's statement that 'you either set moral rules or you develop critical thinking skills' (Holt 2005) reflects a restricted view of available options. It also reflects Holt's understanding of moral guidance as a form of indoctrination or moral training that denies moral agency by seeking to get students to become mere rule followers. This is, of course, an inappropriate educational aim for nurses if they are to be autonomous and accountable practitioners, yet there is a suspicion that some teaching of ethics to nurses takes this form. They say 'moral guidance provided by an educationalist may be considered proper for primary school children, [but] more is expected of both educationalists and students in nursing education' (Holt and Long 1999, p.247). The something more they advocate is the teaching of ethics as a separate subject like any other in nurse education with an emphasis on critical thinking and logical reasoning. These things are important and are to be supported in the pursuit of the autonomous and accountable practitioner, yet neither learning ethics nor philosophical method can take the place of an education that seeks to encourage in students the sorts of dispositions considered desirable, if not essential, for practising nurses.

When they claim, 'The guidance required by students is not moral guidance on how to act, but guidance on how to critically evaluate the beliefs and arguments advanced on ethical issues' (p.247) they distinguish between actions and beliefs as well as between character and reason. Yet, despite the later claim that their approach enables students to undertake moral evaluations of actions (which again is an important skill), it still allows students to view the learning of ethics as an intellectual exercise one step removed from (their own current and future) professional moral responsibility. Once knowledgeable about ethics and philosophical method we may be able to evaluate our actions as wrong or right, as harmful or beneficial, yet we may still choose to act in wrong or harmful ways.

The moral education of nurses

If neither ethics teaching nor moral guidance is sufficient for the development of an ethical practitioner then there seems to be a case for the moral education of nurses. Yet this idea remains slightly odd for, as I have stated, one might reasonably imagine that those charged with the education of nurses already take seriously the development of the character as well as the intellectual and practical skills of the nurse.

Indeed, it might seem odd because it is very often assumed that moral education is of relevance to the general education of children rather than adults and as such remains an issue for teachers in primary and secondary rather than those in tertiary education. Generally speaking, it is true that teachers are likely to have some influence on the moral development of children and young people up to the age of 16 in compulsory education (especially those in primary schools), and on those between 16 and 18 who remain in full time education. The school and teachers will influence how pupils come to view themselves and their relationships with others, whether or not the teachers intend it. Those schools (and teachers) that take seriously the idea that there is no such thing as morally neutral education will take steps to ensure pupils learn not just about core curriculum subjects but also about acceptable moral behaviour. In such schools attempts are made to show in operation, amongst other things, justice as fairness and respect for others. Teachers are expected to behave in ways that demonstrate commonly held values (McLaughlin 2005), so the teacher awards marks to work on the basis of merit of work presented rather than on some personal characteristic of the student, does not victimise or bully pupils, and so on.

These sorts of expectations underpin the values held in high esteem in liberal democracies and form the basis of the moral education of our children. It would be odd to imagine that there should be different expectations of lecturers in higher education. Lecturers who do not exhibit these sorts of characteristics earn our censure because they 'set a bad example'. In other words, it is acknowledged that a lecturer's failure to act in morally acceptable ways has the potential to be a negative influence on students. This supports the view that teaching is not a value-free activity and illustrates that moral education continues beyond compulsory schooling. However, this is not to be confused with indoctrination, the thought of which, as Carr (1991) points out, leads some teachers to avoid their moral obligations to students for fear of being so accused. Thus it is not only the school that provides a legitimate vehicle by which a liberal democracy attempts to educate for citizenship which is, in part, a moral education (Callan 1997; White 1996); that role is also a function of the institution of higher education.

By far the majority of literature on the subject of moral education is concerned with the moral education of children and the implication is that by the time an individual has reached the age of majority the general shape of their moral sensitivities has been established. This concentration on moral education in relation to children is understandable, for it is during the developments of childhood that individuals are thought to be at their most receptive to ideas about how people ought and ought not to behave towards others (and this is precisely why indoctrination is seen as a harm rather than a good in liberal democratic societies). Yet the enthusiasm with which some 18–21-year-olds (the traditional age of students in higher education in the UK) embrace causes they later come to reject is evidence writ large of precisely the sort of receptiveness to moral issues that we hope to inspire in school children. And this receptiveness in 18–21-year-olds suggests that moral education should not be restricted to those in compulsory schooling. While issues in the moral education of 18–21-year-olds (those who might be described as experiencing 'late adolescence') is of general interest, it is with the moral education of nurses who make up a particular group of post-18 students that this book is concerned. As a sub-set of post-18 students, nursing students form part of a group studying in preparation for professional work and it is for this reason that the moral education of nurses is a matter of some import.

Professional work is identified in this book as work that aims to provide benefit to others in terms of particular and specified human goods; what Sockett calls the professional 'ideal of service' (Sockett 1993, p.16). Following Koehn (1994) this category of professional workers includes what are thought of as the traditional professions of medicine, law and the clergy but is extended to those other occupational groups (variously described as semi-professions, vocational groups or similar) with a strong public service ethos such as teaching, nursing, social work, youth work, physiotherapy, occupational therapy and so on. What these groups share is the aim of working for the benefit of individual, as well as public good; and in many cases such workers profess to be engaged in work that furthers the possibility for people to obtain goods which are taken-for-granted as goods as such. But in the pursuit of these other-regarding goods something more than ordinary everyday morality is required if we are right to expect, for example, nurses to be more trustworthy than non-nurses. It follows that those involved in the education of nurses must assume either that nursing students already have a grasp of what counts as appropriate moral behaviour as a nurse or that there is something for students to learn in this respect as they proceed through pre- and post-registration nursing education. The former view presupposes that there is no need for the moral education of nurses because earlier moral education for citizenship has not only been successful but is also sufficient to meet the demands of professional nursing work. The latter view assumes neither of these things and leads to recognition of the necessity for some form of moral education within the framework of nursing education. Pre-registration nursing students in the UK must normally be at least 18 but there is no maximum age for entry onto a nursing programme.[3] This, together with the requirement for continuous professional development, means that nursing students may span the entire age range of the working nursing population. As such to talk of the moral education of nurses is to talk of the moral education of adults and not just of 'late adolescents'.

Professional ethics

The apparent neglect of the moral education of adults is relatively recent for, according to Burnyeat, Aristotle's *Nichomachean Ethics* represents a series of lectures aimed at those young men of good upbringing who already have 'the necessary beginnings or starting points...[that is]... correct ideas about what actions are noble and just' (Burnyeat 1984, p.57). Thus Aristotle was concerned with the moral education of adults, or at least the moral education of those young adults who had already learned something about moral character, rather than with the moral education of children as such. Additionally, there is a significant body of writing about professional ethics from the second half of the nineteenth century. For example, both Emile Durkheim (1858–1917) and Florence Nightingale (1820–1910), albeit from rather different perspectives, highlighted the need for those engaged in professional life to cultivate certain sorts of habits of character.

For Durkheim the development of professional ethics was core to ensuring the increasingly complex modern society of his time could withstand the apparent fragmentary forces of capitalism. As Turner puts it 'Durkheim's major concern...was: how can we find a system of moral restraint which is relevant to modern conditions?' (Turner 1992, p.xiv). In a large part the answer is to be found in the title, *Professional Ethics and Civic Morals*, given to the book published in 1957 containing a series of Durkheim's previously unpublished lectures. For Durkheim, professional moral codes are essential because as he forcefully reminds us 'There is no form of social activity which can do without the appropriate moral discipline' (Durkheim 1957, p.14). Durkheim's analysis remains relevant in the early part of the twenty-first century precisely because in many respects the problems with which he was concerned remain central to civic life in modern liberal democracies and beyond.

Florence Nightingale's concern was born from practical necessity. The public perception of nurses as callous gin-soaked miscreants illustrated so evocatively by Dickens in the form of the Sairey Gamp character in the novel *Martin Chuzzlewit* was a barrier not only to the recruitment of ladies as probationers who would be able to provide care appropriate not only to the needs of the sick but also to the well-being of patients. Nightingale's insistence that probationers needed further instruction in cultivating certain types of character traits reflected her view that the moral education of those ladies to that date was insufficient preparation for professional life (Sellman 1997). In other words, Nightingale took the view that moral education for the professional work of nursing is part of an ongoing development of character that extends beyond childhood.

Education for the practice of nursing

Thus far I have intimated that nursing is both professional work and one of a number of social practices. I have claimed that such work is of a fundamentally moral nature and as such requires that attention be given to the moral education of those who engage with it. I have suggested that while the moral education of those in compulsory schooling may be sufficient for the development of good citizenship it is not necessarily sufficient for professional life in the social practice of nursing. Indeed, in Aristotelian terms, those embarking on a professional career in nursing can be considered as the very individuals who require an education in ethics (what we would now understand as a moral education) in order to move from what may be (more or less) morally acceptable behaviour born of mere habit and obedience to convention towards reasoned ethical action; from merely acting morally to being moral.

And this is necessary precisely because of the extra-ordinary challenges to everyday morality faced by nurses and others working in the health care environment.

Because nursing is a practical activity, nurses must be able to deliver safe and effective physical care, particularly in acute situations, but nursing is more than a mere set of physical tasks. Yet in the UK it seems that many nursing students have a restricted view of the nature and purpose(s) of nursing born of prior experience of working as, for example, a care assistant in a health care environment. Such experience is considered a desirable prerequisite for entry to pre-registration nursing programmes because, amongst other things, it suggests an enduring wish to work with patients. Indeed, it is not unknown for an admissions tutor to advise a potential recruit to get this type of experience before applying to join a nursing course. However, the nature of care assistant work is such that learning on the job will most likely be a form of training rather than an education and it is this that can lead an individual to mistake nursing for those very particular tasks they have been trained to perform. But 'good' nursing requires propositional knowledge (know that) as well as practical knowledge (know how). To these we might add 'know when', and something like this combination is what Aristotle calls *phronesis*, often translated as practical wisdom, being the capacity to know when to do the right thing to the right person in the right way and at the right time (Aristotle 1953). *Phronesis* is Aristotle's practical virtue; it is the virtue by which other virtues (those of the intellect and of the character) are given appropriate expression. Borrowing from McLaughlin (2003a) who uses the term *pedagogic phronesis* to describe the practical wisdom necessary for good teaching, I have claimed elsewhere (Sellman 2008, 2009) that one of the aims of education for nurses and others engaged in professional activities is to make possible, indeed to positively encourage, the development of *professional phronesis* in students and practitioners. This idea encapsulates the notion that while compulsory schooling may aim to educate for citizenship and for everyday *phronesis*, it does not prepare sufficiently for professional life, whereas professional education should strive to educate for *professional phronesis*.

If this is true then it should be clear that professional education must do more than merely teach propositional and practical knowledge; it must educate for professional practical wisdom, this is to say that those involved in the education of nurses must take seriously their obligations in enabling students to develop *professional phronesis*. And this means that one important feature of professional nursing practice is (to paraphrase Aristotle) the ability for an individual nurse to aim at doing the right thing with (or to) the right patient at the right time in the right way and for the right reason(s). Understood in this way it is evident that propositional and practical knowledge (knowing that and knowing how) of itself is insufficient for *professional phronesis*.

Education for *professional phronesis* is a form of moral education. Moral education presupposes that people do in fact have enduring traits of character and that it is both possible and desirable to encourage in students dispositions that contribute to human flourishing while at the same time discouraging character traits that detract from the pursuit of human goods. As such, moral education is education of character as well intellect. In this largely Aristotelian conception of ethics, moral education seeks to ensure that, in the realm of nursing practice, knowledge and/or technical ability is not divorced from associated and inherent values. This is important for nursing as a professional practice, as opposed to say plumbing, precisely because nursing aims at human goods and, therefore, requires more than mere technical mastery and expertise.[4] It is not that moral education is a separate subject to be taught in the way that physiology or ethics may be taught, it is rather that the practice of education per se should not ignore or neglect matters of character. In education for professional life it is necessary that practitioners are encouraged to behave in morally acceptable ways not just because of externally imposed stipulations but because to behave in morally acceptable ways is part of what it means to practise professionally. This suggests that patients are well served if nurses are encouraged to develop those virtues appropriate to the ethical practice of nursing. If this is correct then one legitimate part of the role of the nurse teacher is that she or he should strive to inculcate students of nursing with the virtues of nursing.

The nature of virtue

For the purposes of this book I am accepting a largely Aristotelian account in which the existence of something approximating an enduring character is accepted. On this account a virtue is understood as a general disposition the possession of which leads a person to act, from inclination, in ways consistent with that virtue. This is to say that a person's character is illustrated by the exercise of the virtues. Thus, as Hursthouse (1997) characterises it, a just person acts in ways that are just rather than unjust, a courageous person acts courageously and so on. A virtue may be primarily a moral or an intellectual disposition, although some virtues may not be easily categorised using this particular binary distinction, and the virtue that provides the possibility of unity of the virtues is *phronesis* (practical wisdom). Because this account is no more than a brief outline it leaves much unsaid and thus offers much for which it might be criticised. It implies, amongst other things, that a virtuous person has perfection of character but this suggestion is not intended, for virtue is to be found in aiming at, as well as hitting, the mean. The mean in Aristotle's account is not mathematical because for each virtue the mean is closer to either the deficiency or the excess: so courage is closer to rashness or foolhardiness than it is to cowardice. Aristotle recognised that in order to become virtuous one must aim to act in the right way, in relation to the right person, at the right time and for the right reason. This requires aiming for the mean in respect of any given disposition and in relation to the circumstances in which expression of that particular virtue is necessary or desirable. Thus the virtuous act is an act in the right measure (at the mean) and not an act that reflects either of the corresponding vices of deficiency or excess. Thus while a person may be generally disposed to act in a courageous way, the acts of a courageous person will be different under different circumstances because different virtuous actions are called for by those different circumstances. Moreover, it is not supposed that a virtuous person will hit the mean at every attempt as the fallibility of individuals is accepted. Hence, in at least this one sense, virtue is aspirational. At worst, full virtue may not be achievable, but this does not detract from the value of efforts to live well and in ways that add to the possibility of human flourishing. Even in the absence of full virtue, fewer impediments to flourishing are likely than in the absence of any attempts at virtuous behaviour. The admitted circularity of this argument should not detract from the fact that virtues such as those of courage, honesty and justice are recognisable as virtues.

Harman's challenge to virtue ethics

In this section I will extend the discussion of Harman's challenge to virtue ethics that I have outlined elsewhere (Sellman 2007). Harman

(1999) poses a particularly serious challenge to virtue ethics when he claims that we may be mistaken about the whole idea of character. In his view it is likely that what we take to be character is an illusion brought about by a wish to be convinced by our moral intuitions. In a thinly disguised attack on Aristotle, Harman argues that we should be as wary of our moral intuitions as we have learned to be about our intuitions of the physical world. Wolpert (1992) illustrates how far removed from common sense scientific thinking actually is, and argues that it was the attachment to common sense (that is, our intuitions) about the physical world that prevented the development of science until recent times. Harman claims that if character traits do exist then studies to identify them would not have been so spectacularly unsuccessful. On the basis of this lack of evidence, Harman concludes that what we have is a failure of interpretation; we have fallen into the trap of 'the fundamental attribution error' in explaining actions in terms of permanency of character whereas (he says) the evidence points to the important role of situation in determining behaviour. Noting that character defect explanations of conformity in Milgram's experiment[5] and of failure to assist in the parable of the Good Samaritan are unconvincing and undermined by empirical evidence, Harman proceeds to offer alternative interpretations of the data in which features of the situation are brought to the fore. He concludes that our tendency to seek evidence to confirm our existing beliefs leads us astray in inferring character traits from actions, and in generalising from narrow and context bound regularities in behaviour.

In one example, Harman notes that the myopic person who ignores a colleague when passing at some distance may do so because he cannot see him but is very likely to be considered to have failed in some way as a person; that is, as a failure of character even though it may be the more mundane result of not wearing glasses. Because of this we should not be so hasty to damn others in terms of their character when there may be situational reasons for any 'apparent' character fault. Harman does not deny that people have dispositions; rather he denies that people's dispositions are morally significant in the sense implied by virtue ethics. It is not that people do not want to act courageously, honestly or justly and for the most part, given the situations in which people find themselves, such 'virtuous' actions are possible. If one is usually in a situation in which acting honestly is possible then a disposition to act honestly will *appear* to be part of an enduring character, but if there is no such thing as character and if one's situation changes such that one can no longer act honestly then, in Harman's terms, acting dishonestly cannot be uncharacteristic as such.

Harman's analysis is both situationalist and behaviourist; a point not lost on Kupperman (2001) who provides a response in which he claims Harman misunderstands the nature of character. Kupperman accepts a link between virtue and situation but argues that the virtuous agent is a rare animal indeed. Harman's mistake, according to Kupperman, is to suppose that people of 'full' virtuous character are common, and it is this that leads Harman to assume that character traits do not exist. Further, he notes that Harman's attachment to the 'situationist' approach prevents him from acknowledging what Kupperman considers to be an artificial binary (polarised by the 'personologists') within psychology. In contrast, Kupperman comes across as a moderate and pragmatist insofar as he concedes character as both indefinite (that is, changing over time) and the necessity of an interaction, even interdependency, between character and situation in the ability of an individual to express virtue. He concludes:

> we can be said to know of some people that they are reliably honest...in certain sorts of situations... Even in the case of someone who very noticeably is not always 'the same', there can be some imaginable forms of behaviour that we can be highly confident in not expecting. (Kupperman 2001, p.249)

Kupperman acknowledges that *some* behaviour of *some* people might be unwisely attributed to dispositional character traits (an attribution failure) when it is merely habitual rather than moral (or morally motivated) and as such, these people are unreliable, especially in unusual circumstances. This has the effect of appearing to support Harman's contention that dispositional traits do not approximate permanent features of individual character but remain mere responses to situation. The mistake here is to fail, as Harman does, to distinguish between character traits and simulacra. Further, Kupperman notes the tendency in moral philosophy to ignore the relationship between 'the study of morality on the one hand, and on the other axiology (the study of what are genuinely worthwhile goals or values)' (2001, pp.245–246). This gives rise to a failure to recognise the effects of unfamiliar sets of moral norms within unfamiliar circumstances. For individuals this means a separation between ethical behaviour in normal everyday situations where axiological matters are not at stake and ethical actions in unfamiliar situations where one's values and goals are challenged. If one is operating predominately in the former then it may be relatively easy to establish, or at least approximate, dispositional character traits, but it is within the latter that enduring dispositions of character will be exhibited. Kupperman recognises that there are occupations ' in which normal practice seems to differ significantly from what [a]... person's previous moral training would have led him or her to expect' (2001, p.246). This point is often made in nursing where it is said that the study of health care ethics is necessary for nurses precisely because by becoming a nurse a person enters an unfamiliar world for which experience of everyday acceptable (moral) behaviour provides insufficient preparation for the difficult ethical issues that arise in the practice of health care (see, for example, Edwards 2009; Hussey 1990; Quinn 1990).

Harman is right to doubt the reality of character despite, or even because of, most people's intuitive sense of its existence. It is, after all, the examination of fundamental assumptions about the world around us that philosophy encourages. But for Harman this is more than merely an academic exercise and he is correct to recognise that it may not be possible to prove the existence of character, but that of itself does not prove its non-existence. Nevertheless, he does seek to provide sufficient grounds for us to acknowledge the possibility that we have been misled by our intuition and in this respect he reminds us of the need to remain open-minded about the existence or otherwise of character.

In addition, as Kupperman acknowledges, we are well advised not to neglect the effect of situation on moral behaviour. For even if one is to accept the existence of character virtues, to consider the expression of virtue as immune from the influence of circumstance is to imagine something approximating perfection. Proponents of virtue ethics have long recognised that difficult situations provide a test of character, and some would argue that it is the capacity to exhibit virtue in the face of difficult situations that proves the existence of character. However, Kupperman may be right to note that 'full' virtue may be rarer than we would like to imagine and that therefore few individuals are able to act in the right way, at the right time, for the right reason and in relation to the right person in situations that make the expression of virtue difficult. Perhaps modernity has led us to become complacent about virtue as most of us find we are required rarely, if ever, to put our character to the test. Yet we admire those whose character is tested and not found wanting. Such is the stuff of heroes and many find inspiration in the admiration of those who can act well in spite of considerable difficulties.

Professional virtues

It can be said then that general virtue offers the possibility of guiding normal everyday moral behaviour but seems to provide insufficient grounding for acceptable moral behaviour within the professional practice of nursing. This is not a failure of virtue itself for, as implied in the foregoing discussion, ordinary everyday life (at least in twenty-first century western liberal democracies) rarely provides a sufficient test of character and makes it difficult to distinguish between genuine disposition and mere situation-induced habit. Thus, arguably, modernity fails virtue by not providing sufficient opportunities for individuals to develop a sense of general virtue beyond that required for ordinary everyday living. Working as a nurse involves being confronted with dilemmas for which a poorly developed sense of general virtue provides insufficient guidance for moral action. While many have attempted to fill the resulting vacuum of moral guidance with deontological, utilitarian, principle-based or rights-based ethical approaches, Potter (2002) reminds us that, at best, the application of these moral theories has only ever been partly successful. If general virtue cannot yet compete with the more established moral theories then perhaps a consideration of virtue as it applies to situations beyond the ordinary will offer a fresh perspective. To differentiate between everyday general virtue (that is, the everyday, sometimes poorly developed, sense of virtue that suffices for normal everyday living) and the idea of a form of 'extended virtue' (that is, a well developed sense of virtue that provides guidance for practising nurses), I shall use the term *professional virtue* for the latter.

Clearly, there are problems with the use of this terminology for the notion of 'extended' or 'professional' virtue as I have defined it is merely what others would call virtue. In virtue ethics there is no distinction to be made, one either has a virtue or one does not. And if one does not have a virtue, one can choose to aim for it, can ignore it, or be indifferent to it. This much can be admitted, but in talking about professional virtues I am not attempting to deny this characterisation, rather I am attempting a discussion of the virtues in relation to the professional practice of nursing. It is not that there is necessarily a substantive difference between a virtue and a professional virtue to be debated but it is to indicate that professional practice challenges the expression of virtue precisely because of the contrast between the exercise of virtue in normal everyday life and the exercise of virtue in the challenging world of nursing and health care. There will be other occupations (or practices) for which the expression of virtue is equally challenging and in this respect some similarities between nursing on the one hand and, for example, social work, teaching and youth work on the other will be apparent. But the argument of this book is focused on the practice of nursing and hence any claims made here will not be generalised at this point.

Particular professional virtues

From what I have stated already it would seem that professional virtues are merely extensions of everyday virtues, and in one sense this is precisely what is intended. However such a view provides only part of the story, for it is necessary to take account of the fact that, like everyone else, nurses inhabit a modern and fragmented world. A world in which we occupy multiple roles each of which may require us to exhibit different sets of traits if we are to successfully negotiate our way in life. So, despite the injunction of the NMC (2002a) that nurses must act at all times in ways consistent with the tenets of the nurses' code, a nurse will also adopt different roles at different times and, importantly, not all of these roles will necessarily be compatible. There may be occasions when a nurse will act, while not engaged in nursing, in ways where the expression of a particular virtue is differentiated from the way someone engaged in the practice of nursing necessarily exhibits that same virtue. Additionally, there are traits of character that might be more important in nursing than elsewhere. It may be, for example, important to be meticulous in a particular nursing role but this does not necessarily require that same person to be meticulous when not working as a nurse. Thus there is a sense in which professional virtue is different in both substance and importance from everyday virtue although it is recognised that this is to challenge not only the idea of the unity of virtues but also the idea that a virtue is an enduring disposition. I will return to these issues in various ways throughout this book for they are important challenges that require attention.

In Chapter 3 I argue that nursing is a practice in the sense in which Alastair MacIntyre (1985) uses that term. This means that nurses can choose to engage with nursing in ways that enable the expression of virtue. While it is recognised this would ideally make possible the expression of 'full' virtue which can be extended into, or transferred in from, other areas of nurses' lives, it may be that the best that can be achieved by some nurses takes the form of a weak (perhaps even a modern) sense of virtue. This minimal conception of virtue allows for what I am calling professional virtue and as such offers the individual constrained by the fragmentation of modernity an opportunity to exercise virtue in at least one part of her or his life. Even in this minimal conception, MacIntyre's three core virtues of justice, honesty and courage are given a place of central importance. Some discussion of these three virtues as they apply to the practice of nursing is offered in Chapter 3 but because their expression is relatively uncontroversial I am content to consider the discussion of these three virtues to be a prelude to discussions about the main focus of this book, that is, an examination of the place of trustworthiness and open-mindedness in nursing practice. It is not that other virtues are unimportant; rather it is that trustworthiness and open-mindedness are (relatively speaking) neglected in accounts of nursing despite their importance.

Trustworthiness

The NMC code requires that a nurse must be trustworthy (NMC 2008b) but the trustworthiness suggested by the NMC does not go beyond some elementary notions of financial and material probity in dealing with patients' belongings and in relation to ensuring, for example, that gifts from patients do not lead to favourable treatment for some to the detriment of others. In this conception trustworthiness is little more than an injunction for nurses to practice justice as fairness, yet most nurses will recognise there is more to being trustworthy than this. There is after all evidence of public trust in health care professionals in general (O'Neill 2002) and of nurses in particular, and this is reflected in the public perception that it is scandalous when a nurse betrays public trust. Despite this general recognition that nurses should be trustworthy what this requirement entails is poorly articulated. In this book I make an attempt to provide a preliminary articulation of just what it means for a nurse to be trustworthy. It is not clear that trustworthiness can be properly described as a virtue for reasons that are detailed in Chapter 4 and because of this it is appropriate, I believe, to consider that, in terms of virtue, trustworthiness is best conceived as a professional virtue.

Open-mindedness

It is generally accepted in the health and social care disciplines (and elsewhere) that practice should be based on evidence. This emphasis on evidence-based practice brings with it some problems which, to date, remain unresolved. One of the most pressing, perhaps, is in determining what counts as legitimate evidence, or rather, what evidence the busy health care professional should pay attention to and what evidence should be discarded or ignored. Being open-minded allows for the possibility that there is some evidence that is currently discarded or ignored which should not be; in other words being open-minded about sources of evidence militates against a narrow view of what counts as evidence. And this, as I argue in Chapter 5, is a necessary condition of professional practice. But there is more, for having a general disposition to be open-minded is essential to professional practice precisely because it makes less likely those reactionary tendencies that lead to narrow-mindedness or credulousness. And this makes fulfilling the obligation for each registered nurse to remain up-to-date and competent easier to accomplish, for the open-minded nurse will be aware that not only is what is considered best practice likely to change over time but also that current (possibly cherished) practices may turn out to be wrong or inappropriate. Moreover, open-mindedness is a pre-requisite for *professional phronesis* and if *professional phronesis* is a legitimate aim for nursing education then the neglect of attempts to encourage the appropriate amount of open-mindedness among nurses will be a wilful disregard of a necessary component of professional practice.

Education for professional virtue

For Aristotle, it only makes sense to think about ethics as separate from practical and political life in order to study the inter-relationships and to enable cultivation of the virtues that go to make up attempts to live a good life. This is to be contrasted with the modern tendency of categorisation and fragmentation that leads to ethics being perceived as an academic discipline with its own terminology and nuances that separate it from the everyday practical world in which we live. Where ethics is taught to nurses in this modern sense of ethics as a separate subject then students will and do struggle to make sense of the sometimes daunting theoretical positions of various protagonists. It might be overly simplistic to say that nurses want formulaic answers to pressing practical problems rather than lengthy and complex treatises on, for example, subtle theoretical distinctions between different versions of, say, naturalism or prescriptivism, but given the busy lives of most nurses it is a view that does not stray too far from reality. Thus it is not that the teaching of ethics to nurses is inappropriate, far from it; rather it is that the teaching of ethics to nurses in the modern sense of a subject separated from its practical application is inappropriate.

In Chapter 6 I will say something about how an alternative approach to the teaching of ethics might be pursued but there is much to be said about nursing first and the following chapters will set the scene for that later discussion of the moral education of nurses. Suffice it to say at this point that there is indeed a place for the virtues in the moral education of nurses and some of the reasons for this have been rehearsed in this chapter. Nurses often operate at the margins of human suffering and being exposed to human frailty in ways that few, if any, other occupational groups are, requires that nurses be not only clear about the purposes of nursing practice but also about the need to act in ways that accord with the pursuit of human goods, particularly where achievement of those goods is challenged by the additional vulnerability of being a patient. This requires more than a mere absence of vice in nurses *qua* nurses but, at a minimum, it requires the practice of professional virtue. For some, professional virtue will be a reflection of, or may lead to, full virtue in their lives which would be to fulfil those human goods leading to Aristotle's *eudaimonia* – translated to mean something akin to, 'happiness', 'a good life', 'well-being' or 'flourishing'. This, not unsurprisingly, is likely to be rare in our post-modern age and I should make it clear at the outset that it is not the purpose of the arguments of this book to propose nursing as a way to *eudaimonia*. Nevertheless, such an outcome would not be inconsistent with the primary function of nursing understood here as a response to human vulnerability. The idea that patients are vulnerable is a generally uncontested notion and yet what is meant by expressions such as 'the vulnerable patient' is rarely explicated. Thus there is a need for an exploration of the idea of human vulnerability and it is this that forms the content of the next chapter.

2 Human Vulnerability

In the nursing literature there is a tendency for various groups of clients (or potential clients) to be described as 'vulnerable'. Thus we read of 'the vulnerable child', 'the vulnerable family', 'the vulnerable adult' and 'the vulnerable older person', and more generally we are told of various 'vulnerable groups' in society for whom, as nurses, we are required to be extra vigilant, extra careful or extra observant. If we do not, then these vulnerable individuals or vulnerable groups will suffer or come to some harm from which they have limited resources to protect themselves. Generally speaking to use the word 'vulnerable' in this way is to attach to it a semi-technical meaning in order to denote that individuals thus described are in some way more vulnerable than ordinary people, or *more-than-ordinarily* vulnerable. However this extended use of the word vulnerability is rarely acknowledged, and even less often explained, as being used in a technical or semi-technical sense. Rather it is assumed that it is known what is meant when one or other person or group is referred to as vulnerable: after all we do tend to recognise that the 'vulnerable adult' is an adult who is more likely to come to harm than someone for whom the label would be inappropriate. Those described as vulnerable are perceived to be vulnerable because they appear to be particularly susceptible to harm as a result of either a higher than normal exposure to risk or a reduced, sometimes absent, capacity to protect themselves. For such persons this increased risk of harm is compounded by their reliance upon others, including institutional others, to protect them in ways that are, generally speaking, unnecessary for ordinary individuals.

But this is already to identify a difficulty in using vulnerable as an adjective in this semi-technical sense because ordinary people are also vulnerable. Indeed, vulnerability is part of the human condition and to say that some patients are vulnerable fails to distinguish between ordinary and extraordinary vulnerability. Furthermore, to say that some people are vulnerable is to imply that others are not: yet the idea of a non-vulnerable person or patient is unsustainable. We are all vulnerable and our individual vulnerabilities are related to our own particular circumstances at any point in time. Or to express this slightly differently, we may all share certain common features of vulnerability but we all differ in some of our specific individual vulnerabilities because of the particular situations in which we find ourselves at any given time or place. The extent of our vulnerability is not constant for we may be less or more vulnerable on any given occasion dependent upon a range of factors only some of which are amenable to our individual influence.

If all people are vulnerable then it must be true that all patients are vulnerable, and if all patients are vulnerable then there is little point in describing some individual patients or groups of patients as vulnerable for that is merely to state the obvious. The best that might be said is that to use the phrase 'vulnerable patient' is to use a form of shorthand on the assumption that common understandings exist about what such a claim actually means. Thus 'the vulnerable adult' may be shorthand for 'an adult who is at high risk of a particular sort of harm or set of harms as a direct result of her or his specific vulnerability at a particular point in time' or for 'an adult who is vulnerable in ways that are beyond what we normally understand as ordinary human vulnerability'. This reinforces the idea that all clients are vulnerable but that the vulnerability of some clients is such that they are more likely to suffer harm from particular and predictable sources. On this account one of the responsibilities of the nurse is to know both what those sources are and how to offer suitable and appropriate protection, insofar as such measures are possible and reasonable. It also emphasises the fact that to be vulnerable is to be vulnerable to something.

It is worth noting at this point that this is not a claim for a single 'technical' definition of vulnerability. Rather it is to note that current use is imprecise and ambiguous. Nurses from different fields of nursing (as well as nurses from within the same field of nursing) may indeed have different ideas about which individuals or groups are or are not vulnerable. However there is a generally accepted idea that there are individuals who are particularly vulnerable, that is, at risk of certain sorts of harms and/or abuse and that this vulnerability is one of the things that identifies an individual as a client.

The idea that some clients require more protection than others is evident in many nursing accounts. The list of vulnerable adults would include, among others, individuals with learning difficulties, those undergoing cytotoxic chemotherapy for cancer, those with mental health problems and those in intensive care.

In this chapter I explore the meaning of vulnerability both in general terms and in the context of health care in the attempt to bring some clarity to the use of the term in nursing. I make a distinction between ordinary and extra-ordinary vulnerability and claim that it is appropriate to consider patients, by definition, to be *more-than-ordinarily* vulnerable. Further, I claim that it is helpful to understand nursing as a response to the additional human vulnerability that comes with being a patient. Being *more-than-ordinarily* vulnerable compromises the possibility for human flourishing in ways that being ordinarily vulnerable does not. If nursing actions are predicated on ideas of minimising the effects of patients' additional vulnerability or of reducing patients' vulnerabilities to particular and knowable risks of harm then it would be true to say that one legitimate aim of nursing is the promotion of flourishing for *more-than-ordinarily* vulnerable persons.

All people are vulnerable...

That human beings are vulnerable is a self-evident truth. It is to state the obvious to note that all biological entities are at risk from harm precisely because of the nature of the environment in which biology is possible. Despite some quite remarkable powers of adaptation all living organisms operate in an environment where dangers exist. The dangers to which human beings are exposed can be categorised in different ways but any classification of the risks of harm must take account of those that are inter alia physical, psychological and social, as well as those that are internal or external. Thus vulnerability is part of the human condition and harm may come from many sources. If Maslow (1968) is to be believed, we strive to satisfy our most basic needs for safety and security at the expense of all else (assuming food and water to be part of safety and security) in the attempt to minimise our vulnerability. But we are never entirely free from the possibility of being harmed no matter how far we organise our environment(s) to protect us from the vicissitudes of everyday living.

However, our vulnerability is not a constant. We are vulnerable in different ways at different times to different sorts of threats of harm. We are able to take more or less effective actions in the attempt to reduce our vulnerabilities as we negotiate our way through our lives. When we are newborn we are arguably at our most vulnerable for at that time our dependency on others to protect us from harm is absolute. If we are fortunate enough to develop and grow in ways that we have come to understand as normal then we reduce our dependency on others for protection in ways that mark out our transitions on the way to adulthood and maturity. But this is not a mere linear progression as, on the way, we will inevitably have occasion to fall back upon dependency in some form and we may ultimately return to a state of dependence in our final years. This characterisation of our journey through dependency on others for protection from harm is merely illustrative. For each of us will experience the journey in an individual and subjective way. The threats to our survival and flourishing will be different in detail from those of our contemporaries as well as from those of our elders and our successors. And our responses to those threats will be individual insofar as we are all unique.

In addition, and despite our quest to be autonomous and independent, it is apparent that any individual is limited in her or his scope to reduce her or his vulnerability, and even this is dependent upon the social and political environment in which the individual is living. Ultimately, our efforts to minimise our vulnerability are dependent upon the general good will of others, in both formal and informal ways. Under normal circumstances, we trust others not to take advantage of our vulnerabilities. I have already suggested that we are especially vulnerable as infants. Other times when we might be said to be particularly vulnerable include: during sleep, when we are distracted, following some intense physical exertion, and when we find ourselves with a degree of physical incapacity. While it is true to say that at such times we are more vulnerable than when we are awake, when we are not distracted, when we are not exhausted, and when we are physically fit respectively, it remains the case that these examples describe parts of our ordinary everyday vulnerability.

This ordinary vulnerability is, in part, a function of the uncertainty with which we live and this uncertainty poses risks to our continued survival and to our possibilities for flourishing. We cannot be certain that those things on which we depend will be there for us tomorrow. Nevertheless, we tend to assume that if we go about our everyday lives following the normal social conventions and rules then we will end the day relatively unscathed. But there is no certainty about this and, as the Stoics[6] remind us, if we come to rely on the idea that all will go well for us (that is, that we are in some sense *invulnerable*) then our expectations will not only expose us to disappointments but will also leave us ill-prepared to deal with the harms that befall us. Hence to ignore our inherent vulnerability is ultimately counterproductive as it makes us more rather than less vulnerable; or rather it renders us susceptible to fears about the possibility of losing those things that we most value. And if we value the wrong things (that is, those things that we might easily lose, those things that are most susceptible to harm) then our vulnerability is increased and our sense of safety compromised. Seneca's[7] remedy for this possibility of what we might now call angst is to make sure that we do not place value on those things for which we cannot offer protection and to be realistic about the uncertainty of our lives. That is, we should not always expect things to go well for us but recognise instead the possibility that things may not turn out as we hope. If we are able to accept a realistic conception of our place in the world (that is, that things are neither arranged for our benefit nor that the natural order of things is likely to be just) then we will free ourselves from angst and in so doing render ourselves less vulnerable, particularly to those things about which it is foolish to consider we have any control.

The danger in following this advice is that we might come to live our lives too passively, accepting all that befalls us with equanimity. In accepting events as inevitable we become more vulnerable if we fail to take elementary and simple measures to protect ourselves. It would be folly to think that protective actions are futile because of a view that 'what will be will be'. If I were to walk in the road rather than on the pavement in the belief that what will happen to me today will happen regardless of any action I might or might not take to protect myself then it would appear that I have put myself at risk unnecessarily because by walking in the road I have increased the chances of being harmed. I have become more vulnerable. Luck may play a part in my ability to get to the end of a day unscathed but it is not just a matter of luck. It is rather a mixture of, amongst other things, luck, judgement and social and political trust.

Luck

Some would consider it good fortune indeed to have been born in this time and in this place rather than in some earlier time or in some other place. But if it is the case that luck is the reason for our survival to date this is not to say that we should be content to continue to rely solely on luck. In our striving for certainty and safety we continually battle against mere luck and some even suggest that we make (at least some of) our own luck. To rely solely on luck would be to accept a fatalistic view of our existence, and our continued survival as individuals as well as as a species would be sorely tested. If we are mere captives to fortune we remain at the mercy of events and this leaves us without any way of predicting which actions might protect us from harms.

Thus in some respects we have luck to thank (or curse) for our current situation and we will inevitably remain vulnerable to the sorts of uncertainties about which we cannot offer protection or a defence. In short we will always be vulnerable to certain sorts of threats of harm. But, as noted above, vulnerability is not a constant and the extent to which a given individual is vulnerable will vary. Moreover, given that there are certain things to which an individual will always be vulnerable, there are other things to which that same individual will be more or less vulnerable and the degree of that vulnerability will change over time and place. This is to say that while I may be in the wrong place at the wrong time (a common expression of the role of luck in our lives) and suffer harm as a result, the amount of harm I experience may be determined by a range of factors only some of which I may be in a position to influence.

Pedestrians walking on the pavement do get injured by motor vehicles on occasion (when, for example, a driver looses control of his vehicle or is incapacitated in some way) and we tend to think that those harmed in such circumstances are particularly unlucky. In contrast some particular others will feel themselves lucky indeed to have escaped harm for they might have been in that same spot at the 'wrong' time but for some seemingly random event that resulted either in their early or late arrival at the location of an accident.

Judgement

We can and indeed we do strive to reduce both the role of luck in our lives and our vulnerability with varying degrees of success. Our individual successes occur in response to the sorts of threats we can guard against; that is, the sorts of harms about which we can be reasonably confident in our predictions. This requires the use of judgement. Thus we can be reasonably confident that, under normal circumstances, if we walk on the pavement rather than in the road we will avoid being hit by a motor vehicle. This is the sort of prediction we rely upon when going about our daily business but in being only reasonably confident we must allow that there is no absolute certainty of our safety.

Generally speaking we do act so as to reduce our vulnerability. Actions such as walking on the pavement rather than in the road normally have an actual protective effect, although it is quite easy to imagine that not only might there be specific occasions when walking on the road is safer than walking on the pavement but also occasions when walking on the road *in spite* of the risks may turn out to be the safer option. It would, for example, be safer to walk on the road when the pavement is being repaired and a clearly marked walkway has been erected specifically to allow pedestrians safe passage.

However, our vulnerability is not necessarily lessened when we do take protective measures although our perceptions of vulnerability may be changed significantly. Generally speaking, actions that lead to reduced perceptions of vulnerability enable us to proceed with our everyday lives. And this is the case whether or not our actions actually do provide us with (some) protection or whether or not our actions fail to reduce the risks. However, reducing perceptions of vulnerability is not always compatible with human flourishing, as will be illustrated later in this chapter. Nevertheless, under normal circumstances, it would be foolish not to take some protective measures especially those commensurate with a reasonable assessment of the risk versus benefit of taking rather than not taking an action. To walk in the road rather than on the pavement would seem to be unnecessarily risky, although it would turn out to be safer to have walked in the road if, by chance, a lorry had shed its load on the pavement at that moment. It seems to be important for people to reduce their perception of their own vulnerability whether or not their vulnerability has actually been reduced. This is important for to live with a perception of a high level of personal vulnerability may reduce a person's capacity to flourish. Under normal circumstances, then, it would be reasonable to state that one of the motivations of human behaviour, at least in everyday activities, is to seek out actions that reduce one's vulnerability. If we are successful in this then we make ourselves, or at least perceive ourselves to be, less vulnerable.

Recognising those things that we can reasonably protect ourselves from and taking actions so to protect ourselves (and our important others) requires the use of judgement. But in recognising these things we also by default recognise that there must be things which we have limited ability to effect. While there remain judgements to be made about some parts of these things there is much that we must take on trust. Ultimately we must come to judge how far we can trust in the social and political institutions that surround us.

Social and political trust

In some matters our predictions are predicated on a notion of social trust that we hope others will respect. We anticipate that on the whole drivers will not deliberately steer their vehicles onto the pavement and we trust they will maintain their vehicles in a state of roadworthiness such that they will not suddenly mount the pavement as a result of mechanical failure. There are, of course, social and political structures that provide us with some basis for this trust. It is a general social expectation (as well as a legal requirement at least in the UK) that drivers drive with 'due care and attention' and while the majority of drivers continue to recognise some mutual benefit in driving in socially responsible ways then our trust is well founded. In addition, there are regulatory powers that have the effect of assuring us that our trust is generally warranted. Again in the UK at least, motor vehicle owners are required by law to ensure their vehicle is maintained in a roadworthy condition and there are penalties for failure to comply.

It is worth noting here that social and political trust should be understood as operating within both formal and informal institutions that may exist in either physical or virtual forms. In the UK the Department for Transport is an example of a formal institution with a physical presence; whereas the UK Highway Code is formal but has no physical presence (other than in its written form). The Highway Code, road signs, road markings and so on together make up a social institution insofar as motorists tend, on the whole, to accept and observe these 'rules of the road' for their own safety and for the safety of others, including pedestrians.

Risks of harm

I have argued that being vulnerable is part of what it means to be human. I have suggested that those who are able do, under normal circumstances, take steps to reduce or minimise their vulnerability to the sorts of harms against which it is reasonable to suppose actions can have a protective effect. Thus, while I may come to physical harm by being hit by a moving vehicle I can (and do) reduce the likelihood of such harm by, in general, walking on the pavement rather than in the road. Similarly I protect myself from psychological (and potentially physical) trauma by avoiding situations that are anxiety provoking. And while there remain differences in the way individuals view risk such that what one person may perceive as dangerous or anxiety provoking may not be viewed this way by another, it remains the case that our assessment of risk tends, on the whole, to lead us to act in ways that we believe will protect us from harm. Hence we do tend to act so as to reduce or minimise our vulnerability while recognising that some of the reduction in our vulnerability stems from our trust in the social and political institutions upon which we rely to protect us from the sorts of harms that lie beyond our immediate control.

I have noted here that there are different sorts of risks of harm to which we are vulnerable. In terms of our ability to act so as to reduce our vulnerability it is possible to distinguish three different types of risks of harm.

Type 1 risks of harm

Those risks of harm against which an individual has the opportunity to take actions that have a reasonable chance of providing some protection. So walking on the pavement normally reduces the risk of harm to individual pedestrians from road traffic.

Type 2 risks of harm

Those risks of harm against which an individual must rely for protection (such as is available) on the actions of others. This may be a reliance on individual others or on some form of institutionalised others. So the pedestrian is protected by the individual other in the form of the driver who drives with sufficient care and attention, as well as the institutionalised others in the form of various social or political institutions that have been developed for the purpose. Thus in the

UK the risks of harm associated with motor vehicle use are reduced by institutionalised regulations. The Highway Code, road markings, traffic signs, MOT testing, seat belt laws and so on, all serve to reduce the general likelihood of harm.

Type 3 risks of harm

Those risks of harm against which an individual is, generally speaking, powerless to protect her or himself regardless of the actions of others. Harms that occur as a result of unexpected or unanticipated events (what insurance companies tend to describe as 'acts of God') which allow only limited scope for effective action would fit this category. The earthquake that destroys a road causing damage to cars and injury to occupants is the sort of event to which we are vulnerable but against which we are, generally speaking, defenceless.

While this categorisation imposes an artificial order it does serve two purposes at this point. The first purpose is to offer a counter to any Stoic tendency toward fatalism. It allows this by providing a guide by which we might determine whether an action we wish to take has a reasonable chance of reducing our vulnerability. So if I am concerned about a particular risk of harm and I believe that risk to be a type 1 risk (as described above) I might be more tempted to act to protect myself than if it were a type 3 risk. The second, and more important, purpose is to illustrate both the scope and the limitations of our individual and/or institutional interventions in any attempt to reduce or minimise our vulnerability.

The categorisation has only limited application for it will be immediately apparent that each of the three types of risks of harm identified above are likely to be influenced by aspects of one or both of the other two. In addition, the roles of luck, judgement and trust will have a significant effect. So while I may judge it reasonable to walk on the pavement in order to reduce my vulnerability, when the lorry sheds its load it may well be a matter of luck that I remain unharmed (or of ill luck if I am harmed). But by continuing to believe that walking on the pavement will, on the whole, reduce my vulnerability I am placing my trust in a number of institutions including those that regulate the use of motor vehicles, and this trust is a matter of judgement. The judgement that I should continue to place my trust in these institutions is reinforced daily by my experience that most vehicles do seem to be maintained in a roadworthy condition and that most motorists drive in socially responsible ways. There may come a time when I begin to believe that a significant number of motor vehicles are not being maintained, or that many drivers are flouting the general rule that the pavement is for pedestrians. Should this happen I would need to revise my judgement about the protective effect of walking on the pavement because my trust in the social and political institutions will have been compromised.

...but some people are more vulnerable than others

I noted earlier that when we are asleep, when we are distracted, when we are exhausted, and when we are physically incapacitated we are particularly vulnerable but that this is a normal part of our general everyday vulnerability. However, any one of these examples has the potential to become debilitating and as such would lead us to become vulnerable in ways that are beyond our normal everyday vulnerability. People debilitated in these ways are *more-than-ordinarily* vulnerable. The notion of being *more-than-ordinarily* vulnerable is to be distinguished from being more vulnerable as part of our ordinary everyday vulnerability.

On this account those whose mental development does not match their physical development might be considered *more-than-ordinarily* vulnerable; those who are likely to fall asleep at any time of day while undertaking any activity would be *more-than-ordinarily* vulnerable; and those who become so distracted that it interferes with their normal everyday functioning are also *more-than-ordinarily* vulnerable. Thus we recognise that not only are we more vulnerable at some times within our ordinary vulnerability but also that we may become *more-than-ordinarily* vulnerable. And it is reasonable to suppose that when we require the services of health care workers in general and of nurses in particular we are or have become *more-than-ordinarily* vulnerable.

The purpose of differentiating between these two senses of vulnerability is twofold. It provides a basis for establishing the meaning of the semi-technical, but often unarticulated, way in which the term vulnerable is employed to categorise particular groups and individuals, and it also serves as a reminder of our shared human frailty. Despite our everyday vulnerability we do retain a capacity for flourishing as human beings. It is true that there are many threats that pose a risk to our well-being and it is also true that these threats are threats precisely because of our ordinary human vulnerability, but our ordinary everyday vulnerability does not, of itself, prevent our flourishing. Ordinary people with ordinary vulnerabilities do flourish in the world in spite of the myriad risks of harm to which we are all exposed (although this is not to imply, as Carel (2009) reminds us, that those who are *more-than-ordinarily* vulnerable cannot or do not flourish). Of course, this is an artificial dichotomy that is, at least to some extent, socially constructed and its imposition can lead us to forget our own essential vulnerability. To describe some individuals and groups as vulnerable suggests that others are in some sense invulnerable or non-vulnerable – a claim that cannot be sustained. What follows from this is the recognition that our vulnerability is a matter of degree and that when we say we are vulnerable what we mean is that we are vulnerable to something. We are ordinarily vulnerable just so long as we retain the capacity to act in ways that offer us some protection against the everyday harms to which we are all vulnerable (albeit that we must at the same time take some things on trust). We are *more-than-ordinarily* vulnerable when, for whatever reason, that capacity is compromised. So our vulnerability is not merely a function of the extent of our exposure to harm but it is also a function of our capacity for self-protection.

A person who has their protective capacities intact and who is exposed, for the most part, to type 1 risks of harm (those against which we have the possibility of taking protective actions by and for ourselves) might be said to be ordinarily vulnerable and hence have the potential to flourish. This is to say that, if such a person chooses to pursue the good life then there would seem to be little in the way of external obstacles that would prevent them from so doing. Whereas, a person whose protective capacities are compromised and who lives with the continual threat of type 2 risks of harm (those against which she or he must rely on the actions of others for protection) will have more obstacles to overcome if they are to flourish. This is particularly the case either where those others cannot be trusted to provide some degree of protection or where the individual perceives that the social and political institutions cannot be relied upon to act for the public good. People whose vulnerability is exposed to type 3 risks of harm (those against which there is little human intervention that can have an effect) have even less opportunity to thrive regardless of their own capacitates for self-protection. And being *more-than-ordinarily* vulnerable compromises the possibility of human flourishing in ways that being ordinarily vulnerable does not.

People who are or who become recipients of health care in general and nursing care in particular can therefore be considered, at least in general terms, *more-than-ordinarily* vulnerable because their exposure to type 2 and/or type 3 risks of harm has increased, and because their capacities for self-protection are compromised. The further the balance of types of risks of harm moves towards types 2 and 3 risks for any given person the greater the threat and likelihood of harm precisely because they are *more-than-ordinarily* vulnerable. Thus all patients can be considered as *more-than-ordinarily* vulnerable. This is not to deny differences degree in being *more-than-ordinarily* vulnerable and as such some patients will be at greater risk than others just as some ordinarily vulnerable persons are more at risk than others.

Patients as vulnerable people

Current descriptions of certain patients or groups of patients as vulnerable remain unsatisfactory for at least two reasons. One reason is the ambiguity that can arise when different understandings of the term-in-use collide; a second takes the form of a recognition of the different susceptibilities of individual patients.

Ambiguity in use

Looking in from the outside, current use of the adjective seems to include just about everyone. It spans the entire age range of human existence; as in 'the vulnerable child', 'the vulnerable family', 'the vulnerable adult' and 'the vulnerable older person': as well as different patient groupings; 'the vulnerable ITU patient', 'the vulnerable cancer patient' and so on. While all these groupings may share common features of vulnerability what the descriptions fail to do is to say anything about what these patients or groups of patients are vulnerable *to*: hence the potential for ambiguity. By way of illustration, health visitors consider the 'vulnerable child' as one who is, in older terminology, 'at risk' (Appleton 1994) and this is quite a different meaning from that used when claiming that children should be thought of as a 'vulnerable group' when it comes to being research subjects (Royal College of Nursing (RCN) Research Society 2003). While it is true that the meaning of the vulnerability in each of these examples *can* be determined by the context, it nevertheless remains a distinct possibility that confusion and misunderstandings could occur, especially in the context of interprofessional working and the globalisation of health care. This suggests that the term vulnerable is insufficiently precise; it may have some value in generally parochial and rather vague understandings but it does not identify the source of the risk of harm. A person described as vulnerable is usually at risk of harm from specific and predictable sources.

Individual patients, different susceptibilities

Recognising the inadequacy of the adjective 'vulnerable' and replacing it with more accurate terminology does not of itself remove the problem of imprecision. For even if it is accepted that all patients are *more-than-ordinarily* vulnerable it remains true that not only are individual patients more susceptible to harm in different ways and at different times but also that some patients are more vulnerable to particular risks of harm than others. Generally speaking, but not invariably, individuals who are unconscious are likely to be more vulnerable than those who are conscious, and the same is probably, but not always, true for people with cognitive or physical incapacities. Despite variations it is nonetheless possible to say with some certainty that the unconscious patient is *more-than-ordinarily* vulnerable because to be unconscious is to have an absent capacity for self-protection in some very specific ways. Thus we know that a patient who is unconscious is at risk of harm from a blocked airway and thus protection from this specific and predictable source of harm is an important and necessary action for a nurse to undertake.

Clarke and Driever's account

Clarke and Driever (1983) attempt to develop an account of patient vulnerability drawn largely from social and developmental psychology. Their account is located within a framework of what are claimed to be the central concepts of nursing theory. Fawcett puts it thus: 'A consensus now exists that the central concepts of the discipline of nursing are person, environment, health, and nursing' (Fawcett 1983, p.4). In fact, this statement represents only one particular view (a predominately North American view) of the central concepts of nursing and as such cannot be held to provide the global consensus claimed. Nevertheless, it is a claim that permeates the work in the volume in which Clarke and

Driever's paper appears. As a result their discussion of vulnerability is constrained and their account partial.

Clarke and Driever argue for a construct of vulnerability for nursing 'based on the subjective perspective of the individual [and a]... perceived transaction between the capabilities and environmental situations that determines the individual's wellness–illness status' (1983, p.210). In other words, their claim rests upon the assumption that vulnerable people are vulnerable *because they perceive* themselves to be vulnerable; and on the idea that such vulnerability is a function of an individual's *perception* of a lack of capacity to protect themselves from the external environment. They further claim the subjective nature of vulnerability has a psychosomatic effect on the health of the individual. Those with a perception of themselves as having a high level of vulnerability lack the confidence to face the world and tend to react to their environment in ways that are 'not conducive to healthy development' (p.211). Whereas the 'individual whose self-perception is one of low vulnerability... tends to develop into a healthy, resilient, competent person' (p.211). This highly speculative claim rests, as they rightly acknowledge, on an extension of the claims of psychology. Thus, for Clarke and Driever, a low perception of vulnerability is a prerequisite for flourishing.

They also suggest a need to distinguish vulnerability from risk and they do this by conceptualising vulnerability as subjective and risk as objective. While superficially attractive their failure to offer a defence of this characterisation of risk leaves the idea unsubstantiated. Consequently their claim that 'Risk, the objectively assessed potential transactions between individual capabilities and challenging environmental situations, is determined by others' (p.212) is unconvincing.

Despite this they firmly locate vulnerability as a subjective experience and risk as the objective and external threat to well-being. Their construct allows them to suggest that the function of nursing is both to act on the external environment (to reduce the risks) and/or to assist the individual patient to feel less vulnerable (for example, by using techniques developed from psychological theory to reduce the individual's perception of their own vulnerability). In this way it is claimed that nursing can affect the transaction between the patient's vulnerability and their exposure to risk, thus enhancing the patient's sense of well-being.

They are right insofar as they draw attention to the fact that to be vulnerable is to be vulnerable *to* something and their recognition of vulnerability as a function of the interaction between the person and the environment is important. It is also correct to say that one proper function of nursing is to attempt to provide a safe environment in which patients can be nursed and while this might reduce the risk of harm to an individual patient it does not necessarily reduce that patient's *feelings* of vulnerability. The emphasis on reducing patients' feelings of vulnerability is misguided although in doing so Clarke and Driever unwittingly illuminate the significant difference between perceptions of vulnerability on the one hand and actually being vulnerable on the other. However in characterising vulnerability as purely subjective they are unable to account for those whose capacity to articulate their subjective experience is in some way compromised. Thus the three main claims of Clarke and Driever's account require further consideration.

Claim 1: risk as objective and external

While it is true to say that risk can be objective and external, neither is a necessary condition. Risk can be also subjective and internal: physical, psychological, emotional, and so on. A physical internal risk may come from naturally occurring bodily changes including, for example, an aneurism, a cancerous growth or general degenerative changes. A psychological risk might come from, for example, holding the false belief that there is a risk of imminent collapse of a building. Assuming there to be no physical evidence for this, and assuming that the structure is not built above the site of some natural 'disaster waiting to happen' (for example, hidden and unknown mine workings), then it would be difficult to say, in this case, that the perception of risk is either an objective or an external phenomenon.

Claim 2: vulnerability as purely subjective

Clarke and Driever state that: 'the subjective quality of vulnerability relies on perception, the knowing and understanding brought about by awareness gained through the senses' (p.213). Thus they make no allowance for the possibility that someone who is unable to know or understand their vulnerability can be vulnerable. In so doing their account fails to recognise that many recipients or potential recipients of nursing practice do not have the full range of capacities necessary to articulate the subjective experience of vulnerability, for example, those with severe mental and/or physical disability; those in a coma; infants and those with Alzheimer's disease. It would be unusual to claim that people in such states should not be considered vulnerable. Vulnerability is not just a subjective experience. It is a part of our nature to be vulnerable, whether or not we recognise the fact, it is only a subjective experience when we recognise or pay attention to it. It would be strange to say someone is not vulnerable just because they are not experiencing a sense of vulnerability when, for example, they are merely walking along the pavement, for all sorts of eventualities may befall them. We are all clearly vulnerable for it is part of our nature to be vulnerable even when we do not perceive ourselves to be vulnerable.

Thus while it may be important for ordinarily vulnerable people to have a low perception of their vulnerability if they are to flourish in the world this is neither without constraints nor is it significant in the same way for *more-than-ordinarily* vulnerable persons. For ordinarily vulnerable persons to have a perception of vulnerability that is so low as to be virtually absent is to tempt them to begin to feel 'invulnerable', and, as suggested earlier, to feel 'invulnerable' is to run the risk of actually increasing vulnerability. Similarly for *more-than-ordinarily* vulnerable persons a sense of 'invulnerability' is generally speaking incompatible with human flourishing. Moreover, attempts to reduce feelings of vulnerability in those *more-than-ordinarily* vulnerable persons whose capacity for recognising their vulnerability is compromised to a greater or lesser degree will be of questionable value, and, in some cases, might not be possible at all.

Claim 3: the patient will feel less vulnerable

If I have understood them correctly, Clarke and Driever claim that nurses should adopt psychological interventions to make their patients feel less vulnerable on the grounds that feeling less vulnerable is a good thing. However, as suggested above, there is no reason to suppose either that feeling less vulnerable necessarily equates to being less vulnerable or that getting patients to feel less vulnerable is necessarily an appropriate aim of nursing practice. It is possible to imagine nursing interventions that succeed in enabling a patient to reduce her or his feelings of vulnerability while at the same time increasing the likelihood of harm.

While it is true that people do wish, in general, to reduce their feelings of vulnerability and while it may be that in some instances in nursing this may have some therapeutic value, there may be instances where reducing feelings of vulnerability is unhelpful or even counterproductive. The competent adult surgical patient may feel less vulnerable once she or he understands the safeguards that exist to protect patients while under general anesthesia. But apart from the suspicion that this may be merely an exercise in anxiety reduction the patient will still actually be vulnerable during an operation. The patient in a coma being nursed in an intensive care unit will actually be less vulnerable when certain protective procedures and protocols are observed but is unlikely to feel less vulnerable while she or he remains unconscious. The patient who is unable to judge the extent of risk from certain sorts of behaviour or threats would not be well served by the nurse who led them to believe they were less vulnerable than they actually are. The patient who believes she or he can fly would better served by being encouraged to feel more rather than less vulnerable when about to launch her or himself from the third floor of a building.

Thus merely to accept that helping people to feel less vulnerable is a good thing is not a position that can be sustained. Encouraging people to feel less vulnerable may lead to foolish risk taking and consequently compromise human flourishing. If, for example, I am persuaded to believe that I am in some sense less vulnerable than I really am then my assessment of the risks of everyday activities may lead me to act in ways incompatible with my capacity to flourish. To return to an earlier example, if I choose to walk in the road rather than on the pavement in the belief that I will not be harmed by this action then I will have increased the likelihood that I shall be harmed. It may be that for a while luck and the care of others will be sufficient to allow me to continue walking the road without being harmed. I might find myself only walking on roads with slow moving traffic, or on roads that are sufficiently wide to enable motorists to swerve and avoid hitting me. But while this may appear to validate my belief that walking in the road is a safe option it is unlikely that my luck will hold out indefinitely. When I find myself on a busy or narrow road it may be that a motorist travelling at speed around a blind bend is unable, because of other factors outside of her or his control, to avoid hitting me. Thus sooner or later I shall be harmed and my supposed reduced vulnerability will prove to have been a folly.

So the claim of a therapeutic reduction of the perception of vulnerability may apply where perceptions of vulnerability get in the way of human flourishing, as in the case of the earlier example where that perception was based on a false belief, but it cannot be assumed that it will be a good thing in all situations. From this it should be clear that judgement is required to ensure that in any therapeutic attempt to reduce feelings of vulnerability an individual's sense of vulnerability remains consistent with human flourishing. To do otherwise is to effect rather than avoid harm. This, it seems is no simple task for it requires a normative ontology absent in the account offered by these authors.

Patients as *more-than-ordinarily* vulnerable people

To state that all patients are vulnerable is to do no more than recognise our common human frailty. It would be more accurate to say that patients are *more-than-ordinarily* vulnerable.

One aspect of those described as *more-than-ordinarily* vulnerable (as in 'the vulnerable adult', 'the vulnerable child' and so on) is that such individuals are perceived by nurses as not only at risk of harm because of an increased exposure to type 2 risks of harm but also, in some cases, because of their reduced or absent capacity to recognise when they are falling victim to the activities of abuse and/or because of their reduced or absent capacity to look after their own interests if they become the victim of the activities of abuse.

This distinction is important and is explained further. As a competent adult I am vulnerable in ordinary everyday ways. As such I may fall victim to, for example, an unscrupulous financial advisor who might choose to exploit my trust in the social institutions that I anticipate will provide some measure of protection from exploitation. I may be reassured by a claim by the financial advisor that he is a member of some guild of financial advisors. It is quite likely that I will accept this claim at face value on the grounds that I believe there to be such bona fide organisations designed to protect individuals from rogue traders. If it turns out that there is no such guild and that I come to recognise that I have been exploited then this will confirm my capacity to recognise, albeit too late, that I have been duped. In addition, and because I am a competent adult, I have the capability to find out how best to go about seeking recompense.

That I might not have taken all the steps available to me to protect myself from such exploitation in the first place may have been the result of a naïve trust in the system of regulation of financial advisors and the worst that might be said is that I should have checked to see if she or he was indeed a member of a bona fide financial services regulatory authority. My failure to do so illustrates both my vulnerability to type 2 risks of harm and the interdependence between type 1 and type 2 risks of harm. There is a question that arises here in relation to the reasonableness of my actions of self-protection. I have said that type 1 risks of harm can be categorised as offering the opportunity to take actions which might have a reasonable chance of providing some protection. I have also claimed that judgement is a necessary component of deciding which actions to take. Such judgement is an essential constituent of practical wisdom in the Aristotelian tradition. The point here is that the judgements I make in relation to actions are dependent upon, amongst other things, my experience of trust to date in the social institutions that I take to function as protective to avoid harm to individuals. Those who are in recipient of nursing practice are not always in a position either to make judgements about protective actions or to know when they are being exploited.

Nurses and protection of clients

I have suggested that one of the responsibilities of the nurse is to be able to provide some measure of protection for clients who are by definition *more-than-ordinarily* vulnerable and who have both a reduced capacity to protect themselves from type 1 risks of harm and an increased exposure to type 2 risks of harm.

The reduced capacity for self-protective actions increases a client's dependency on others to act on her or his behalf. Thus the client comes to rely on the actions of others for protection from ordinary everyday risks of harm and on institutional protection from type 2 risks of harm. This dependency is, of itself, an additional type 2 risk because the client is left to trust that those others have her or his good as a primary consideration. If those others do not have the client's good as a general aim then the client remains not only *more-than-ordinarily* vulnerable to the activities of abuse in general but also *more-than-ordinarily* vulnerable to the activities of abuse of particular others; others in whom trust is placed to offer protection from harm. This is one reason why it is necessary for those charged with the protection of clients to have certain sorts of dispositions, dispositions that are consistent with the protection and flourishing of *more-than-ordinarily* vulnerable people.

On this account protection of patients' particular vulnerabilities is an essential feature of nursing practice. Protection is necessary because patients are *more-than-ordinarily* vulnerable in both general and specific ways. To return to an earlier example, one general feature of being unconscious is an inability to maintain one's own airway. Thus protecting an unconscious patient's airway is a standard feature of nursing practice. However, there may be particular characteristics of a given individual patient that makes them susceptible to other *additional* harms as a result of being unconscious. If these characteristics are such so as to be identifiable without recourse to extra-ordinary means then the nurse would be failing in their duty of care not to take these individual characteristics into account when planning and implementing care for that particular patient. It requires recognition of the unusual as well as knowledge of the general. If the unconscious person is harmed because the nurse failed to take cognisance of the unusual but knowable then she or he has failed in her role as protector of the patient. For the unconscious patient, my competence to provide care rests not only on my knowledge of potential and predictable risks of harm but also on my capacity to recognise the specific as well as general vulnerability of a given patient and to act in suitably protective ways.

If it is the case that one of the functions of nursing in general and of individual nurses in particular is to protect clients from harm then any actions that restrict the flourishing of *more-than-ordinarily* vulnerable persons is fundamentally inconsistent with the practice of nursing. This seems an obvious point and an oft-stated intention. Yet while there seems to be a high level of public trust in nurses the fact is that not only do some nurses sometimes act in ways that result in harm to individual clients but also that the UK regulatory body for nurses believes it necessary to publish guidance on protecting clients from harm (NMC 2002b). Moreover, this guidance is primarily aimed at the protection of clients from the activities of abuse of nurses. The phrase 'activities of abuse' is taken to mean any activity or group of activities, whether deliberate or not, that results, or is likely to result, in harm to an individual or group of individuals. Abuse in this sense is taken to include those harms that result in 'physical', 'sexual', 'psychological', 'financial or material' abuse as well as in 'neglect and acts of omission' (Department of Health 1999, p.8).

In a publication entitled *Practitioner-Client Relationships and the Prevention of Abuse* the Nursing and Midwifery Council state that

'Registered nurses…have a responsibility to protect clients from all forms of abuse' (2002b, p.7). Nevertheless, the stated aim of the publication is 'to protect the public by helping *to prevent the abuse of clients by practitioners*' (p.3; emphasis added). In effect, the document outlines the nature of professionally acceptable practitioner–client relationships in the attempt to ensure that *more-than-ordinarily* vulnerable people are not subjected to activities of abuse by nurses. While it may be reassuring for the public to know that the regulatory body for nurses takes the protection of *more-than-ordinarily* vulnerable people seriously it may at the same time raise questions in the public domain about the general trustworthiness of nurses. I take it to be important that nurses should be trustworthy and I will pursue questions about trust and trustworthiness in relation to the practice of nursing in Chapter 4.

At this point it is sufficient to note that there is a professional recognition that those who are the recipients of nursing care are *more-than-ordinarily* vulnerable and that it is necessary for nurses to be ready and willing to adapt their practice to ensure that *more-than-ordinarily* vulnerable clients are protected from abuse. I want to go further and claim that this 'protective' function of nursing is fundamentally related to human flourishing insofar as without such protection the ability of an individual to flourish is compromised.

The guidance expects nurses to act in certain sorts of ways (that is, in professional rather than unprofessional ways) in order to protect clients. In the UK nurses are accountable to the NMC and are required to practise in a way that is consistent with the tenets of the NMC code (NMC 2008b) – this requirement is also expressed in nursing codes across the globe. But it would be an impoverished account of nursing if it were assumed that nurses act in protective and professional ways only because nursing's regulatory bodies require it. It is true that a nurse's actions are required to be generally protective but it is also assumed that a nurse should be generally disposed to act in protective ways. The nurse who is disposed to act in protective ways is to be preferred to the nurse for whom acting in a professional way requires a conscious decision to act against inclination. Nevertheless, merely being disposed to act in a protective way is insufficient to ensure clients are protected from harm. What is required is that these 'protective' dispositions are cultivated and more will be said about the development of 'protective' dispositions in Chapter 6.

Nurses are vulnerable too!

The discussion thus far has concentrated on what it means to be vulnerable as a recipient of health care in general and of nursing in particular. From what has been said it might be inferred that nurses are in some way not as vulnerable as everyone else, and elements of the idea that nurses are 'special' in the sense of being able to withstand the sometimes harrowing demands of caring for *more-than-ordinarily* vulnerable people do seem to exist in the minds of the general populace. There are those who, once they see for themselves the sorts of things that nurses are required to do, express their own inability to do those same things. Of course, this is to generalise from mere anecdote and in some cases these sentiments may have more to do with a sense of gratitude or a mistaken idea of what nurses and other health care professionals can achieve, but it does nevertheless point to a need to say something about nurses and vulnerability.

It should be clear that nurses are ordinarily vulnerable just like everybody else. Indeed nurses, like all other health care professionals and like all other people, are just as likely to become patients, and it is not unknown for the experience of being a patient to lead some individuals to want to become nurses.

There is evidence to suggest that nurses are one of a number of occupational groups who suffer harm as a result of high exposure to particular occupational hazards. For nurses these hazards include, but are not limited to: back injury (RCN 2002); burnout (Payne 2001); physical assault, threatening behaviour and verbal abuse (Winstanley and Whittington 2004); workplace violence (Anderson 2002); HIV and AIDS (Munodawafa, Bower and Webb 1993); hepatitis (Rogers, Savage and Cowell 1998); cytotoxic drugs (Griffin 2003); insufficient staffing (Humm 2002); substance abuse (West 2002); needlestick injury (Davis, August and Salome 1999); and being stalked (Parish 2000). Thus, nurses are vulnerable to identifiable and predictable sources of harm although in some cases the recognition of increased risk may lead to protective behaviour – one example of the positive benefits of perceptions of vulnerability. Nevertheless, nurses would appear to be more at risk of coming to harm from these, and other, sources than many other occupational groups: possibly at greater risk than other health worker groups. However, in spite of this increased exposure to risks of harm nurses should not necessarily be considered *more-than-ordinarily* vulnerable because nurses' capacities for self-protection are not, as a general rule, compromised.

For the purposes of the present discussion the vulnerability of nurses might be usefully categorised thus:

- nurses are exposed to particular occupational hazards

- nurses witness the *more-than-ordinary* vulnerability of others on a daily basis.

Nurses are exposed to particular occupational hazards

Hospitals are not particularly safe places. The concentration of disease and illness combined with the necessary use of antibiotics leads to a colonisation of harmful infective organisms (many of which are especially virulent and in some cases antibiotic resistant) within many clinical environments. That this is recognised is witnessed by the generally accepted practice of advising immuno-compromised patients to keep away from hospitals wherever possible. The vulnerability of nurses (and other health care workers) to infective agents was graphically illustrated by the quarantining of Canadian nurses exposed to the severe acute respiratory syndrome (SARS) virus during the outbreak in 2003. Hence it is true to say that those who work in hospitals are more likely to come into contact with particularly virulent types of pathogenic organisms than are people who do not work in hospital-type health care environments. However, this does not necessarily mean that hospital nurses are more vulnerable to the risk of harm posed by exposure to potentially harmful organisms. Apart from the fact that there are policies and procedures designed to protect hospital workers in general there is evidence that in those clinical areas recognised as places of high risk the likelihood of harm is diminished as protective practices become the normal mode of operation (Rogers *et al.* 1998). It seems that nurses who work in areas not usually considered high risk may actually be at greater risk of harm precisely because of a reduced perception of risk. For example, nurses working in dialysis units recognise that many of the patients will be carriers of hepatitis, and because of this recognition practice tends to be in strict accordance with universal precautions. Universal precautions are a standard set of guidelines for dealing with bodily fluids on the assumption that all bodily fluids might carry potentially harmful organisms. While adopting universal precautions is considered to be the essence of good practice it is clear that many nurses working outside identified high-risk areas do not conform to the guidance. Paradoxically, this appears to have the effect of placing them at greater risk of harm.

Similarly, nurses working in mental health units are acutely aware of the potential risk of physical harm from violent incidents. Training in the management of aggression and techniques of de-escalation is helpful to mental health nurses with the aim of recognising and defusing potentially violent situations. This perception of being vulnerable to physical harm by virtue of working with clients with mental health problems equates to the identification of a type 1 risk. The individual nurse can take self-protective actions to reduce the likelihood of harm (of course, it is also a type 2 risk of harm as there are institutional protective actions taken at least in in-patient facilities). In contrast, general nurses (with some notable exceptions such as those working in emergency departments) tend to expect fewer violent incidents despite the increase in reported incidents of violence to hospital staff (Winstanley and Whittington 2004). Hence the perception of not being at risk may increase the vulnerability of nurses. One thing that might be said, then, is that nurses are more vulnerable to certain sorts of risk of harm just by being nurses because working as a nurse brings with it a number of risks; risks to which those who do not work as nurses are not exposed. However, because, generally speaking, nurses are not compromised in their capacities for self-protection they remain, at least for the most part, ordinarily vulnerable albeit with an increased exposure to type 1 risks of harm.

Nurses witness the more-than-ordinary vulnerability of others on a daily basis

The expression 'bearing witness to suffering' is common in some accounts of nursing. It is noted as a factor in, amongst others, accounts of the experiences of nurses working in emergency departments (Malone 2000) and in accounts of palliative care nursing (Boston, Towers and Barnard 2001). Malone notes that in the nursing literature vulnerability is most often considered to be essentially negative (something to be avoided or prevented) but there are, as Carel (2009) notes, positive aspects to vulnerability that should not be ignored. One form of a positive approach to vulnerability is expressed by Daniel as 'a trait to enjoy; for through it, humans celebrate the authenticity of what it is to be human' (Daniel 1998, p.191) and later she says 'Vulnerability is a vehicle for practicing authentic nursing'. This use of the idea of 'authenticity' betrays the existential origins of the approach and its proponents argue against the attempts of nurses to distance themselves from the suffering of patients. On this account to practise nursing while distancing oneself from the suffering and vulnerability of patients is to nurse 'inauthentically'. Those who subscribe to this view consider it necessary for each nurse to acknowledge her or his vulnerability as this is essential for good patient care. As Daniel puts it: 'if we deny the opportunity to participate in vulnerability, we deny the opportunity to participate in humanness which then permits us to practice dehumanizing acts' (Daniel 1998, p.191).

Whether or not this is true, it is accepted that to bear witness to the vulnerability of others is generally stressful. In being ordinarily vulnerable like everyone else some, but not all, nurses will succumb to the effects of the stress this constant exposure to the suffering of others brings with it. And, like everyone else, the manifestations of stress will follow the general patterns of stress-related disorders. Burnout is considered to be common among nurses:

> It affects the physical and mental health of the nurse and may carry costs for the employing organization through absenteeism, staff conflict and rapid turnover... Burnout may also affect the quality of nursing care provided to patients and their families. (Payne 2001, p.397)

And it is the last point here that is of particular significance, as anything that impinges on the ability of a nurse to provide protection adds to the increased vulnerability of patients. Interestingly, proponents of the 'nurses need to embrace their own vulnerability' approach claim that becoming more involved with patients' suffering can reduce the likelihood of burnout.

Nurses working in palliative care might be supposed to be amongst those who will most often bear witness to the suffering of others. Yet it is not clear that palliative care nurses come to any more harm than other nurses. One reason for this may lie in recognising the risks of working with people who are dying. Once the risks are identified actions can be taken to minimise the potential of those risks to cause harm, although it should be recognised that this effectively amounts to an acceptance of the idea that nurses do need to become comfortable with their own vulnerability if they are to be in a position to provide professional nursing to those in their care.

Nurses and human flourishing for patients

One consequence of providing protection for *more-than-ordinarily* vulnerable persons is that it enables human flourishing. Hence, human flourishing is a legitimate end of nursing. For while ordinarily vulnerable people are able to flourish despite the risks of harm to which we are all subjected there are additional obstacles to flourishing for *more-than-ordinarily* vulnerable people. In providing protection from the additional risks of harm that being *more-than-ordinarily* vulnerable brings nurses are helping to remove or at least reduce those obstacles that have the potential to restrict the capacity for human flourishing amongst clients. Of course, as Carel (2009) points out, illness (and the vulnerability that comes with it) does not of itself mean that flourishing is restricted, for it is the case that for many individuals the experience of illness brings about a dynamic shift in self-perception of vulnerability and may lead to revelations of previously unrecognised strengths and capacities for flourishing in ways that lay dormant prior to the illness.

Nevertheless, the protection of patients is a legitimate function of nursing wherever the flourishing of *more-than-ordinarily* vulnerable persons might otherwise be compromised. This does, of course, require an account of human flourishing and this will be the subject of Chapter 3. But regardless of the nature of human flourishing it should be clear that those in receipt of nursing care, the *more-than-ordinarily* vulnerable, are vulnerable to obstacles that get in their way of flourishing precisely because they are patients. If this is true then whatever else is taken into account when decisions about care and/or treatment are made it is important that nurses attempt to ensure that it contributes to, rather than detracts from, that patient's capacity to flourish. Of course the detail on this does depend on what is understood by human flourishing but in principle the force of this position is strong. To express this differently, one legitimate role of the nurse is to ensure that the actions of others (including professional others) do not unnecessarily obstruct the flourishing of *more-than-ordinarily* vulnerable persons.

3 Practices and the Practice of Nursing

Nursing is a complex occupation that continues to defy simple definition. In this respect at least nursing shares similarities with other professional occupations (such as teaching, medicine, physiotherapy and so on) where concern for human betterment is at the heart of professional aspirations. It may be that this definitional problem is more acute for nursing than it is for those occupational groups that can point to some centrally important aspect of their practice: education is central to the practice of a teacher; for a doctor it is the diagnosis and prescription of treatments; for a physiotherapist it is such things as manipulating joints and muscles, performing chest physiotherapy and so on. Nurses struggle to identify such centrally defining activities for it is the case that nurses do many things: nurses educate; some nurses diagnose and prescribe (at least in some instances); and many nurses undertake physiotherapy-type tasks. Moreover nurses often undertake these 'specialist' activities in the absence of the 'specialists'. That is to say, that nurses are the only group to provide a continuous 24-hour presence for patients and consequently find themselves doing whatever needs doing at times when 'specialists' are unavailable (although there are, of course, limits to this as nurses are reminded in their codes, for example, Nursing and Midwifery Council (NMC) 2008b, Canadian Nurses Association (CNA) 2008, American Nurses Association (ANA) 2001, to practise only within their sphere of competence). In meeting the needs of patients, nurses are the only group unable to define what they do as limited to specific and particular roles. For example, with the exception of those occasions when there are reasons for a physiotherapist or an occupational therapist to assess a patient's ability to self-care, whenever a patient needs assistance with toileting it is a nurse who is will be summoned. When a patient needs to have a wound redressed, the physiotherapist, the doctor, the social worker and others will call on the nurse. Doctors, physiotherapists, social workers, teachers, occupational therapists and others would not normally consider such activities to be part of their role. Yet, outside of normal office hours, it is generally the case that nurses are expected to do many of the things these other professionals would do were they present. The reverse is rarely true.

Of course, these examples reflect only the stereotypical impression of nursing as a hospital-based and medically-oriented activity. As intimated in the introductory chapter, nursing encompasses a wide range of activity in a bewildering variety of institutional and community settings. This adds to the difficulty in getting to the nub (as it were) of nursing. Nevertheless, some discussion about the nature of nursing is a necessary part of the argument of this book and is essential to this particular chapter in which I pursue the claim that there is benefit in understanding nursing as a practice in the technical sense in which Alasdair MacIntyre uses the term.

I made the claim in Chapter 2 that nursing is concerned with enhancing the flourishing of *more-than-ordinarily* vulnerable persons. In this chapter I make the further claim that, as a consequence of working towards the flourishing of *more-than-ordinarily* vulnerable persons, nurses who engage with nursing as a practice (in the MacIntyrean sense) are, themselves, enabled to flourish as human beings. Of course, these claims must be considered against both the concept of a MacIntyrean practice and the idea of human flourishing. Thus I begin this chapter with an outline of the nature of MacIntyre's concept of a practice and his account of human flourishing. For MacIntyre, rational capacities play a central role in human flourishing and this seems unnecessarily to exclude some *more-than-ordinarily* vulnerable persons. Thus I take it as necessary to extend MacIntyre's notion of human flourishing in order to take account of *more-than-ordinarily* vulnerable persons.

Following these discussions I return to the claim made in Chapter 1 that any attempt to categorise nursing as a science is fundamentally misconceived. Despite the fact that many people think they know what it is that nurses do and/or what nursing is, a history of (presumably) unsuccessful attempts to define nursing testifies to the difficulty of the task. Thus I do not set out to define nursing as such for that task has eluded far more accomplished scholars. Rather, my purpose here is to offer some considerations of the nature of nursing and to note, in particular, some of the reasons why nursing cannot be a science. I will argue that understanding nursing as a MacIntyrean practice in response to human vulnerability allows for the inclusion of the idea that nursing is centrally concerned with human flourishing which, as I suggested in Chapter 2, is a legitimate end of nursing. As such, then, nursing as a practice in which cultivation of the virtues is centrally important is presented as an alternative to the increasingly voiced, but mistaken in my view, idea that nursing is a science.

Practices

I have elsewhere claimed there are advantages in understanding nursing as a practice in the very specific sense that MacIntyre adopts when using the term 'practice' (Sellman 2000, 2010). Here I draw from those earlier accounts to restate and expand the claim further. For MacIntyre (1985) a practice is a form of human activity where possibilities exist for individuals to move towards a good life. His is a teleological vision of a good human life in which individuals might engage with a range of complementary practices which includes engaging with the traditions of those practices. Such engagements would, as a consequence, reduce the fragmentation of individual experience that has become the hallmark of modernity. In other words, MacIntyre offers a vision in which those individuals who engage with a practice (or with a set of practices) enhance the possibility of human flourishing. For it is by engaging with a practice that the goods internal to that practice become available; it is where the virtues are encouraged and have the opportunity to flourish, and it is where some refuge from the fragmentation effects of late modernity might be found.

Before beginning a discussion of practices in the sense in which MacIntyre develops the term it should be noted that his vision of practices is set within a sociology whereby the idea of tradition and the idea of individual narrative complete the story. Hence, while practices are perhaps the first essential components of a good human life, practices do not of themselves represent sufficient conditions for a good life. This is to say that he takes it to be necessary that if there is to be any sense of unity in the idea of human flourishing, practices are to be recognised as only one component, for it is the case that all three aspects (practices, traditions and individual narrative) are necessary if any sense of unity of human experience is to be realised. On this account to engage in a single practice might contribute to, but would not be definitive of, human flourishing. With this in mind I will now turn to an examination of the idea of a practice as defined by MacIntyre.

MacIntyre uses the term practice to refer to:

> any coherent and complex form of socially established cooperative human activity through which goods internal to that form of activity are realized in the course of trying to achieve those standards of excellence which are appropriate to, and partially definitive of, that form of activity, with the result that human powers to achieve excellence, and human conceptions of ends and goods involved are systematically extended. (MacIntyre 1985, p.187)

In order to clarify he uses the example of chess. Chess is a game that only offers internal rewards when played in the 'proper spirit' rather than when played solely to win: although to win by playing with respect for the spirit of the game will be an excellent achievement. To win by playing in a manner that ignores the spirit of the game is to forfeit the possibility of the internal rewards available only from playing in the 'right way'. And playing in the right way requires inter alia paying attention to the rules and traditions of the game, as well as playing with respect for the level of sophistication to which players of excellence have brought the game. To play well is to engage with the game in such a way as to pursue excellence in playing chess.

This emphasis on the availability of internal goods is crucial to the idea of a practice as MacIntyre conceives it, as the internal goods of chess are only available to those who engage with chess (or with some similar species of game) as a practice, whereas external rewards might be obtained in myriad other ways. This is to say that to receive cash for playing chess would be to receive an external reward and an external reward of this type can be achieved in numerous other ways; for example, by winning a lucky dip, by selling groceries or by being in paid employment. Some critics have taken this distinction between internal and external rewards to be a separation but this is to mistake MacIntyre's purpose. MacIntyre does not say that internal and external goods are mutually exclusive, nor does he claim they are necessarily separable, rather he claims that one of the features of a practice (and one that distinguishes an activity as a practice as such) is that those engaged with the practice have access to the internal goods in a way that those not engaged with it do not.

In his later work MacIntyre (1988) refers to 'goods of excellence' and 'goods of effectiveness' rather than to internal and external goods. By so doing, Knight (1998) suggests MacIntyre avoids some of the difficulties that follow from attempts to separate internal from external goods. Like internal goods, goods of excellence are those goods that are only available to the individuals who participate in a practice as a practice, whereas goods of effectiveness can be obtained elsewhere and relate to, for example, organisational or institutional goals. MacIntyre notes that there is an inevitable tension between institutions on the one hand and practices on the other. Institutions necessarily place an emphasis on the goods of effectiveness for it is only by, for example, maintaining a viable financial base that an institution can function in the modern world. And if practices are to survive at all then they need the security the institution provides, especially if the practices operating within that institution are practices that are not wealth producing. So farming, which is wealth producing, may share some of the goods of effectiveness with the institutions under which farming is currently made possible. Whereas nursing is less likely to share in the general idea of goods of effectiveness and, if the institution in which nursing takes place fails to value the goods of excellence, nursing will be hard pressed to survive as a practice. This is to say that not only are practices dependent for their very existence on institutions but that they are also vulnerable to the internal and external forces that affect the institutions themselves. The institution may serve inter alia to protect practices but practices cannot remain immune from external influence. If the institution comes under pressure to reduce its costs then expensive (that is, non-wealth producing) practices will be expected to adopt, at least, some aspects of, the goods of effectiveness and will be forced either to accept cuts in funding or find ways of producing income. While the goods of effectiveness are not necessarily incompatible with a practice there will be a point at which, if the goods of effectiveness become the major focus of activity, the practice will have become so corrupted that it is no longer identifiable as a practice as such. That is, it will no longer offer the goods of excellence to those who participate in its activities.

There remains the problem of how we are to come to recognise internal goods if those goods are not obvious to us before we understand an activity (such as chess) to be a practice. MacIntyre addresses (but does not explain) this as follows. If an adult already immersed in chess as a practice wishes to initiate a child into playing chess as a practice then it is likely that the child will need to be 'bribed' to play in the first instance – MacIntyre suggests in his example this might take the form of the external reward of sweets. Chess is a difficult game in so far as it requires a good deal more of a player than many other games and it is not clear why a child would want to engage with chess as a practice rather than as just another game. However, if the child begins to recognise that there is something in this game of chess that is appealing beyond the promise of the external reward of sweets then MacIntyre would say that the child has begun to engage with chess as a practice. As the child becomes engaged with chess as a practice then she or he will come to recognise that access to these internal goods (those goods which are not otherwise available) is dependent on playing in ways that are consistent with chess as a practice. To play solely in order to win is to reduce the possibility of achieving those internal goods. And while winning by cheating is possible the point of chess is not merely to win but, if winning is to be an aim, to win by excellence in playing the game.

From this we might suppose that MacIntyre is suggesting that we do not necessarily set out to become engaged with activities as practices. In the first instance we may be motivated by external goods or by immediate satisfactions and it is only as we become aware of the possibility of internal goods that we start to participate in activities as practices as we recognise the value of those activities as practices. This is not to say that all activities are, or have the potential to become, practices and one of the criticisms of MacIntyre relates to the problem of 'evil practices', that is activities which would appear to fit his definition yet be generally harmful. In his defence his concept of a practice is set out against a sociology whereby the purpose of a practice is to enable human good. Thus any activity that has evil ends cannot, in MacIntyre's terms, be a practice. In addition, while there may be internal satisfactions to be had for some individuals engaged in 'activities of evil' the fact that those satisfactions can be neither equated with virtue nor transferred with any consistency to other practices that go to make up the good life debars them from being practices as such.

I have previously pointed out that the ability of people to recognise chess as a practice in the sense that MacIntyre uses the term suggests that the concept is one that is a recognisable part of human experience (Sellman 2000). However, his choice of chess as a paradigm case has provided some ammunition for his critics. Miller for example, takes MacIntyre to task for failing to distinguish between what Miller terms 'self-contained' practices on the one hand and 'purposive' practices on the other. In the former category he places chess because its *raison d'être* consists entirely in the internal goods achieved by the participants' (Miller 1994, p.250) and he contrasts this with those practices 'which exist to serve social ends beyond themselves' (p.250). He insists that MacIntyre's failure to distinguish between these two specific and fundamentally different types of practices is a fatal flaw because the vision that MacIntyre develops from his premise of a practice comes from the self-contained rather than the purposive practice. All that is claimed from the example of chess fails to recognise the additional complexity that purposive practices reveal. In the real world of purposive practices the internal goods are observable and measurable by those external to the practice itself.

Miller considers purposive practices as having socially constructed ends and nursing can clearly be placed in such a category. However Miller goes on to say that it is the ends of the practice that can be judged in terms of excellence by those not actively engaged in the practice itself. He provides an example from medicine and he appears to say that a practice is likely to be deformed by those engaged in it if there is no external accountability. He suggests by way of illustration that:

> the medical community [may] come to attach special weight to the capacity to perform certain spectacular operations whose long term efficacy is doubtful – the practice has fallen victim to professional deformation. A good practice here is one whose standards of excellence are related directly to its wider purpose. (1994, pp.250–251)

The final sentiment expressed in this passage would seem to be consistent with MacIntyre's thesis but Miller appears to have failed to perceive that the valuing of an activity within a practice makes it neither an internal good nor, necessarily, a standard of excellence. MacIntyre would, I think, say that all practices necessarily have forces within and out with them that make such deformations a distinct possibility. Whether or not they succeed in corrupting (or deforming) the practice will only be determined in retrospect, and according to MacIntyre, it is necessary for a practice to be in good order if it is not to succumb to the corrupting influences of the institution; and a practice in good order is one in which a majority of those engaged with it do so at the level of a practice.

Miller's claim that, contra MacIntyre, excellence can be assessed from without by reference to the ends of a (purposive) practice needs further consideration. He claims, for example, that for architecture or farming there is a tangible end product about which a person outside of the practice can make an informed judgement. As an outsider I can judge a building in relation to specified criteria and I can assess the quality of a crop of turnips. What I cannot know, unless I have observed the production process, is whether or not the architect or the farmer has engaged with architecture or farming as a practice during production. In Miller's terms it seems that I have no need to know this and yet for MacIntyre this is essentially relevant. Miller wants to judge the ends without reference to means. For MacIntyre this is further evidence of the pernicious nature of modernity. The tendency to imagine that excellence is to be found in objects regardless of the means of production is to confirm the fragmentary nature of our present condition; it is to separate ourselves artificially from our capacities and from our potential to achieve excellence. Nevertheless, MacIntyre's own claim that excellence can only be determined from within the traditions of a practice is perhaps a claim that is too strong. Care, which might be claimed as an excellence of nursing as a practice, is something that can be regarded and judged properly by those not engaged in nursing. The recipients of nursing are perhaps amongst those well placed to judge the standards of care, and this is not just in terms of ends, but also of means. It is not uncommon for patients to be aware of the individual approaches of different nurses and, important as technical skill is, patients will often find the technical ability of nurses difficult to assess but will recognise very readily the difference between the nurse who merely provides care and the nurse with a caring attitude.

Additionally, as Wainwright points out, 'Practices are alike in so far as they meet MacIntyre's definition, but differ with respect to their content, their goals or purposes and their traditions… To try to subdivide practices into different categories would…weaken the concept…'

WHAT MAKES A GOOD NURSE

(Wainwright 2000, p.35). While it might be tempting to categorise practices in different ways, for example, Miller (1994) divides practices into those that are 'purposive' and those that are 'self-contained' and I have previously identified some practices as 'professional practices' (Sellman 2000), this may ultimately be self-defeating. And this seems correct if we accept that MacIntyre uses chess as illustrative rather than definitive, for elsewhere he provides examples of other activities that fit with his definition of a practice. He says, for example:

> Tic-tac-toe is not an example of a practice…nor is throwing a football with skill; but the game of football is, and so is chess. Bricklaying is not a practice; architecture is. Planting turnips is not a practice: farming is. So are the enquiries of physics, chemistry and biology, and so is the work of the historian, and so are painting and music. (MacIntyre 1985, p.187)

And further he states: 'the range of practices is wide: arts, sciences, games, politics in the Aristotelian sense, the making and sustaining of family life, all fall under the concept' (p.188). Hence contra Miller (1994) and my own earlier view (Sellman 2000) it is the similarities in terms of the potential for internal goods that contribute to human flourishing within practices that is important rather than any attempt to categorise practices on the basis of dissimilarities. MacIntyre's reluctance to provide anything like a definitive list of activities that are, or might be, practices is to be seen as a recognition that the production of such a list would be to focus on the wrong things. As it is, students of MacIntyre continue to argue about the grounds for the exclusion of, for example, bricklaying (some say there are examples of bricklaying which would seem to suggest that as an activity it has, at least in some cases, a legitimate claim to be a practice) and there has been a lively debate about MacIntyre's denial of teaching as a practice (see, for example, MacIntyre and Dunne 2002 and Dunne 2003). If I understand MacIntyre correctly it is not that we should endeavour to work out which activities should be classed as practices, let alone expend effort on devising a taxonomy, because this would be to miss the point. To undertake such classification activity would be to fall into the trap set for us by late modernity that leads us to experience fragmentation. Rather we should be involved in the attempt to establish (or re-establish) our engagement with practices if we are to flourish as human beings. However, it should be noted, this will require an element of classification in order that we may begin to distinguish those activities that can properly be regarded as practices from those that cannot.

A list of sorts is, of course, inevitable as claims are made that some particular occupation, hobby, game or other activity is a practice. And the current project to characterise nursing as a practice carries with it a danger that the exercise may ultimately only add to this classification tendency. It has been a surprise to many that MacIntyre denies teaching is a practice, for many teachers find the idea of teaching as a practice to be a helpful and accurate description of what they do. MacIntyre's denial is understandable from the perspective of his grand theory as he finds the act of removing the teaching of a practice from the practice itself symptomatic of what he takes to be the fragmentary tendency of modernity. Teaching and teachers, he says, should not be divorced from the practice into which the novice is being instructed. He explains that a teacher is first and foremost a practitioner, for example, a mathematician who teaches is engaged in the practice of mathematics both in terms of pursuing the excellences of the mathematics and in terms of instructing the 'apprentice' in the appreciation of the internal goods of the subject. While this example is consistent with what he says elsewhere, and in particular with his extended view of induction into social practices in his book *Dependent Rational Animals* (MacIntyre 1999), it only works as an example because it is a simple and subject limited case, it is, in the words of Dunne an 'impoverished conception of teaching' (Dunne 2003, p.357). The example may well work for some subjects and for some types of teaching (that is, discrete and self-contained subjects as typically taught in secondary education) but it does not reflect the experience of many teachers for whom the reality is that teaching is neither subject specific in this way, nor taught in isolation from other related topics. Primary school teaching in the UK is designed to integrate subject specific work in order, we might say, not to compartmentalise subjects unnecessarily. Similarly, while some teachers in higher education have the luxury of single subject practice (philosophy itself might be one such example) many do not, and the teaching of nursing requires an emphasis on the integration of evidence from many disciplines which themselves might, with some justification, make a claims to be practices in their own right. Of course, to these criticisms MacIntyre might reply that such examples merely serve to reinforce his view that modernity has fragmented our experience of the world to the extent that we can no longer understand how it could be otherwise. We should, he might say, recognise within ourselves that it is a mistake to consider 'what is' to be the same as 'what should be'.

Nevertheless, it is true that there is some ambiguity about this within *After Virtue* (1985), the book where MacIntyre first outlines the nature of practices. He appears to use the example of teaching as a practice when he claims, when referring specifically to practices, that justice is a core virtue of a practice. His example of the professor who is obliged to mark students' work on merit and who is therefore exhibiting a proper standard of excellence seems to be a claim that teaching is a practice. And later, and again when talking specifically about practices, he uses teaching as an example when explaining the virtue of patience, 'the patience of...a teacher with a slow pupil' (MacIntyre 1985, p.202) is, he says, an example of how a practice makes sense of a virtue (in this case the virtue of patience). For if not located within a practice there is no answer to the question of the purpose of patience.

But while there may remain disagreement on what is and what is not a practice, and while the categorisation tendency is recognised as a danger, the current attempt to characterise nursing as a practice is undertaken for reasons familiar to many teachers. That is, that many nurses, like many teachers, will find meaning in the idea of nursing as a practice precisely because it offers the potential for the nature of nursing to be captured in a rich conceptualisation which many find absent in existing accounts. But before proceeding with the discussion about nursing as a practice it is necessary to consider what is meant by the term 'human flourishing'. This is necessary for two related reasons. The first is that the claim that nursing is a practice rests, at least in part, on recognising that human flourishing is a legitimate aim of nursing. The second reason is that human flourishing is central to MacIntyre's project and any attempt to understand practices without understanding the relationship of practices to human flourishing is likely to be only partial at best and to misunderstand the importance of practices at worst. For it is by participation in practices that human beings are most likely to find the possibility of flourishing.

Human flourishing
The idea that nursing should be concerned with the well-being of patients is uncontentious and equates with popular conceptions of

human flourishing. However, it is not yet clear what is meant here by the term 'human flourishing'. While recognising that the literature on living well and on what it means to flourish *qua* human is extensive,[8] for the purposes of this book I confine the discussion to MacIntyre's (1999) essentially Aristotelian account in which he emphasises a teleological sociology in which human goods are intimately related to human action, choices and character. However, MacIntyre stresses 'independent practical reasoning' as the capacity necessary for human flourishing and in so doing, he seems to suggest that individuals who have a reduced capacity for independent practical reasoning cannot flourish; although he does say that this is not his intention. In this section I explore some of these issues before suggesting how MacIntyre's description can be extended to include those who, on MacIntyre's account, would otherwise be excluded from the possibility of flourishing.

Macintyre's account of human flourishing

Following Aristotle, MacIntyre (1999) provides a teleological account of human flourishing. Both consider that a good human life is one in which an individual makes proper use of their essentially human capacities in pursuing a life in harmony with those capacities. This requires a life that is both good for the individual as well as good for others. While reminding us that we tend to forget our fundamentally animal nature, MacIntyre argues that the essential human capacity necessary for human flourishing is independent practical reasoning and it is this that distinguishes human from non-human animals. In the pursuit of goods we necessarily make choices and because this is characteristic of human beings it explains why we need to engage with our capacity for practical reasoning if we are to flourish *qua* humans. For we make use of practical reasoning when we choose to pursue one particular good in relation to one particular practice, recognising as we choose that this may be at the cost of failure to pursue other goods. We also recognise our interdependencies insofar as our choices affect others, just as others' choices affect us. Further we have choices to make between projects and, according to MacIntyre, we need the virtues (especially the virtue of independent practical reasoning) if we are to choose well. That is, if we are to choose wisely not only between those projects that contribute to and those that get in the way of our flourishing; but also between competing flourishing-enabling projects.

Noting that we are vulnerable because our projects can be frustrated, he says: 'it is insofar as something tends to interfere with or to be an obstacle to the achievement of…particular goods or of flourishing in general that it is accounted a harm or a danger' (MacIntyre 1999, p.64). Thus we are vulnerable because our projects can be frustrated, and this suggests we can only flourish when we are not prevented from pursuing the completion of our projects. According to MacIntyre: 'What a plant or an animal needs is what it needs to flourish qua member of its particular species. And what it needs to flourish is to develop the distinctive powers that it possesses qua member of that species' (p.64).

On this account it matters a great deal how far a member of a particular species can develop the capacities constitutive of that species; for those who are prevented from realising their capacities will find it harder (in degree related to the severity of the impairment or obstacle) to flourish as members of that species. Thus, because practical reasoning is an essentially human capacity, humans need to be able to develop practical reasoning if they are to flourish. Moreover, it is possible as a matter of empirical fact to recognise those environments that are generally conducive, as well as those environments that are generally hostile, to human flourishing. Hostile environments are those in which not only is human-as-animal survival compromised but also in which there is limited opportunity for the development of human practical reasoning.

Human flourishing and more-than-ordinarily vulnerable persons

From this it would appear that for MacIntyre the flourishing of a human being *qua* human being is possible if and only if an individual has developed the capacity of independent practical reasoning. However, this is surely an impoverished view of human flourishing for, as many nurses and other health care professionals will testify, there are many human beings who evidently do flourish despite an apparent limited capacity for independent practical reasoning. Many such human beings can be described as *more-than-ordinarily* vulnerable as defined in Chapter 2 and in MacIntyre's terms such individuals would not seem to be candidates for human flourishing at all. In his defence he does say that 'It is not…that one cannot flourish at all, if unable to reason' (p.105) but he does not provide an account of flourishing for those who are unable to reason. He does, however, recognise that there are times when we all inevitably fall back on dependency, by which he seems to mean when our capacity for independent practical reasoning is compromised in some way. Additionally, part of his argument for the human need for the virtues revolves around this idea of a natural human tendency to move from dependency towards independence coupled with a recognition that we are all in some sense interdependent because each of us may become dependent during periods when we might normally expect to be independent. Yet, his vision of this 'life journey' fails to recognise that there are those for whom the achievement of fully realised independent practical reason is at best unlikely and on most accounts this fact does not prevent us from considering such persons as human beings who can, at least to some degree, flourish. Moreover, we usually understand such flourishing in human rather than in mere animal terms. At the very least we recognise that there are things that can hinder or help such persons to flourish in whatever limited ways they are capable of flourishing.

If we follow MacIntyre's account, we might say that because humans need functioning independent practical reasoning to flourish *qua* humans then the flourishing of *more-than-ordinarily* vulnerable persons must be of a different order. This would allow for a range of requirements for human flourishing dependent upon a categorisation of human beings as less or more compromised practical reasoners. So we might have, for example, a notion that persons in a coma can only be said to flourish as humans-in-a-coma and not as humans as such. While this has some superficial attraction it creates problems of classification of humans as beings who approximate, to different degrees, an ideal form of being human, that is, the independent practical reasoner. This view seems perilously close to a form of 'moral apartheid' in which differentiated value might exist for different categories of humans with all the peculiar moral judgements (and what are now regarded as morally abhorrent actions) that have accompanied regimes with such perspectives. Apart from anything else, such categorisations of humans would inevitably remain arbitrary and, most likely, capricious. Even MacIntyre would admit, I think, that the independent practical reasoner is to be considered an aspiration rather than a reality; or at least that there exist few fully developed independent practical reasoners. However, there is something we can take from all this in order to extend the concept of human flourishing to include those whom MacIntyre would seem to exclude.

MacIntyre may well be correct in pointing out that the full expression of Aristotelian virtue is only possible for those who have the capacity to exercise independent practical reasoning and while (as far as we know) this capacity is only available to humans, MacIntyre's use of this idea as the quintessential feature of humanity seems to restrict unnecessarily the concept of human flourishing. And this would seem to make possible arguments in support of differential moral status between those who are able and those who are unable to exercise independent reasoning. Hence it seems necessary to extend MacIntyre's account.

Extending MacIntyre's account of human flourishing

Unsurprisingly, MacIntyre's account of human flourishing includes, as a requirement, the potential for purposeful engagement in practices. Such engagement is made possible by the development of the essential human capacity for independent practical reasoning. And for MacIntyre it is engagement with practices that enables the development of virtue. As MacIntyre points out, to engage with a practice it is necessary to recognise the practice has internal goods and to learn that we must cultivate particular virtues if we are to gain access to those goods. This requires a degree of humility and suggests learning is itself a practice for there are undoubtedly internal goods to be had in 'deep' as opposed to 'surface' learning (Marton and Saljo 1976). Further, such internal goods only seem to be available to those who understand learning as something worthwhile in and for itself. It is the case that 'deep' learning encourages the development of the very virtues that enable learning as a practice (and that enable practices in general), including honesty, courage and justice as well as independent practical reasoning. This does seem to raise a problem in explaining the development of virtues by learning to engage in a practice for the latter appears to require the former but this issue cannot be addressed here.

For MacIntyre, independent practical reasoning seems to function much as *phronesis* does for Aristotle. Indeed, those who prefer 'practical reasoning' to 'practical wisdom' as the most appropriate translation of *phronesis* would assume that this is what MacIntyre intends, and on these grounds we might be forgiven for mistaking MacIntyre's independent practical reasoning for Aristotle's phronesis. It seems that, like MacIntyre, Aristotle has in mind only those with the capacity to develop practical wisdom as candidates for *eudaimonia* or human flourishing. If we are to accept the idea that there are those whose potential for human flourishing is compromised or inhibited (those who might be described as *more-than-ordinarily* vulnerable) then we need an account of human flourishing that includes such persons.

I have argued against placing human beings into categories of more or less independent practical reasoners (such as humans-in-a-coma and so on) because this lends itself to justifications of 'moral apartheid'. However, it must be allowed that the capacity for independent practical reasoning will be different for different individuals. As such, we might say that, while independent practical reasoning is a feature of human beings, it is, nevertheless, a feature that varies between and within individuals. This is to say, that not only do individuals have a capacity for independent practical reasoning which may be different from that of their fellows, but also that their capacity for independent practical reasoning may vary from day to day, even from moment to moment, depending upon a whole range of factors. In other words, our capacity for independent practical reasoning is vulnerable to harmful influences from the internal and external world.

On this account, human flourishing can still be couched in terms of a capacity for independent practical reasoning but will require qualification. If we allow that each individual has a particular capacity for independent practical reasoning then we can say that flourishing for a human *qua* human requires that an individual exercise their capacity to the extent that it is possible for them so to do. This means that a person whose capacity for independent reasoning is to some degree compromised can still flourish *qua* human because they can flourish in those ways that their particular human capacities allow. It also means that the care provided by nurses and other health care workers can aim for the flourishing of the *more-than-ordinarily* vulnerable by assisting such persons to realise whatever human capacities they have or by helping to remove obstacles and impediments to the realisation of those capacities.

For those who do not seem to have (as far as we can tell) the capacity for independent practical reasoning at all it is difficult to imagine how they might be said to flourish. Thus there may be some about whom we are forced to say that flourishing is not possible: those in persistent vegetative state, those pronounced dead but kept functioning at a biological level for the purposes of organ donation, and those born without the neuro-biology considered necessary for independent human life would seem to be candidates as humans without the possibility of flourishing. Yet such examples are rare. There are, however, many persons whose capacities for independent practical reasoning are diminished to the degree that they are unable to make the kinds of choices MacIntyre claims necessary for human flourishing, unable, that is, to separate themselves from their desires and thus they remain in a 'childlike' state (at least in terms of independent practical reasoning) in which the satisfaction of immediate desires precludes the possibility of engaging in practices. He says:

> Independent practical reasoners contribute to the formation and sustaining of their social relationships, as infants do not, and to learn how to become an independent practical reasoner is to learn how to cooperate with others in forming and sustaining those same relationships that make possible the achievement of common goods by independent practical reasoners. (MacIntyre 1999, p.74)

Given that a significant number of nurses work with persons whose capacity for independent practical reasoning is challenged and given that nursing work generally aims to enable human flourishing, MacIntyre's account fails to satisfy. If fails to satisfy because his account implies that human flourishing is a case of all or nothing. Yet, for nursing and nurses, particularly for those working with patients whose capacity for independent practical reasoning is (temporarily or permanently) reduced, it is important to understand human flourishing as constituted by the degree to which an individual can exercise her or his independent practical reasoning. In some cases this capacity is compromised (as in, for example, the child with severe learning difficulties) to such an extent that on MacIntyre's account the person cannot be distinguished from non-human animals. On this account not only would the idea of nursing as a response to human (rather than merely animal) vulnerability be undermined but also many of those who are the recipients of nursing practice would be excluded from the possibility of flourishing *qua* humans. In the nursing context in particular it is important to understand that the ability to engage in independent practical reasoning can be partial as this helps to ensure that patients with minimal or compromised rational capacities are understood and cared for as human beings.

From this discussion it can be seen that the virtues have a central place in the concept of human flourishing. In Chapter 1, I described virtues as dispositions forming part of the enduring character of persons. Thus a person's inclination to act in some rather than other ways represents expression of the virtues and this enables us to evaluate their character. This is to say that we can judge the sort of person someone is in relation to those qualities we understand as constitutive of a good human being, and of a human being who can be said to have lived a good life (*eudaimonium*), or to have flourished *qua* human. On this account, a good human being is a virtuous human being; acting in accord with and motivated by the virtues we take to be necessary for a good human life. For MacIntyre the core virtues of honesty, justice and courage are essential to both practices and human flourishing (and therefore for a good human life). Reasons for counting these three virtues as core will be discussed once the case for nursing as a practice has been presented in the next section of this chapter.

Nursing as a MacIntyrean practice
Defining nursing

I have already suggested that, because of the variety of situations in which nursing takes place, defining nursing is not easy. It would appear most people assume that they know both what a nurse is and what a nurse does. For some time the public perception of nurses has been a matter of professional concern to nurses themselves, particularly as many who portray nurses tend to resort to certain well-known stereotypes: the nurse as the selfless angel; the nurse as the smouldering sex symbol; the nurse as the handmaiden of the doctor and so on. These generalised images seem to resist attempts to provide a more realistic picture of nursing. Nevertheless, and despite the acknowledged power of these types of images, nurses and nursing continue to enjoy a high level of public trust and regard.

However, the scope of nursing practice is vast and in general terms it is to be supposed that most people would think of a nurse as someone who tends the sick and (as a social worker colleague was once heard to say) as someone who gives injections. Further it is to be supposed that most people would think first of all that the activity of nursing takes place in a hospital setting but might then concede that it sometimes occurs outside of institutional buildings: in the community and in the homes of those who are in some sense ill. If my suggestion that this is the generally and most commonly held perception of nurses and nursing then we have a problem, not least because the work of many nurses would not be covered in the ideas expressed above.

The range and scope of nursing

It would be to trivialise attempts to define nursing to say that nursing is what nurses do. Nevertheless there is a sense in which it is true because the range of activity of those who can legitimately call themselves registered nurses[9] extends far beyond the range suggested in the paragraph above. Apart from the four separate fields of nursing as regulated in the UK (adult nursing; children's nursing; learning disability nursing and mental health nursing) there are numerous examples of nurses working in diverse and not immediately obvious nursing roles. This breadth of activity in which nurses engage challenges any simple definition of nursing. Perhaps the most enduring and most often quoted definition of nursing is:

> The unique function of the nurse is to assist the individual, sick or well, in the performance of those activities contributing to health or its recovery (or to a peaceful death) that he would perform unaided if he had the necessary strength, will or knowledge. And to do this in such a way as to help him gain independence as rapidly as possible. (Henderson 1966, p.15)

Many have since suggested that Henderson's definition is insufficiently comprehensive and alternative definitions appear from time to time. One slightly more recent attempt describes nursing as:

> The use of clinical judgement in the provision of care to enable people to improve, maintain, or recover health, to cope with health problems, and to achieve the best possible quality of life, whatever their disease or disability, until death. (RCN 2003, p.3)

It might be supposed that the differences between these two definitions would be more striking given the gap of nearly 40 years in their publication. As it stands, the RCN definition seems to have been largely an exercise in rewording although the addition of 'clinical judgement' does give voice to the modern idea of nurses' autonomous professional action.

The rise of the idea of nursing as a science

It is generally supposed that Florence Nightingale was the first nurse to take seriously the idea that empirical data can be used to underpin nursing practice. Thus we might identify Nightingale as the originator of evidence-based practice in nursing. Nevertheless, to those who might further claim Nightingale as the originator of the idea of nursing as a science we can point to her insistence that nursing is an art (Nightingale 1867). Debates about the nature of nursing have exercised the minds of nursing scholars since Nightingale's time and it is not clear that all that much progress has been made for, at the present time, not only is it that the idea of nursing as a science appears to hold a dominant position but also that the ideological gap between those who take nursing to be a science and those who think it an art appears wider than ever.

There have been numerous attempts to refine Henderson's definition and/or to come up with a new and more comprehensive definition in the pursuit of a set of words that captures the essence of nursing. Broadly speaking these attempts have followed a general pattern of what might be called 'the prevailing approach' of any given period. In Nightingale's time the debate focused upon arguments for and against state registration. Interestingly it was Nightingale who held out against state registration on the grounds that it would reduce nursing practice to the lowest acceptable standards.[10] During the 1980s and the early part of the 1990s there was a penchant for models, theories, meta-theories and conceptual analyses of nursing or of aspects of nursing in the search for a theory that might once and for all articulate the true nature of nursing and might also establish nursing as a legitimate and scientific discipline in the academy. These activities drew variously (and one might say arbitrarily) from a range of established disciplines (sociology, psychology, biology, physiology, philosophy and so on) in the attempt to provide a systematic approach to nursing knowledge and theory. Often these attempts arrived at similar sorts of conclusions, for example, about the need to regard patients as bio-psycho-socio-beings who require holistic nursing.

This activity might well be characterised as a nascent academic discipline struggling to develop a knowledge base that it might claim as its own. There seemed to be a prevailing belief that if enough of this type of theorising activity (particularly of the rigorous and scientific sort) were to be undertaken then there would emerge the sort of theory of nursing that many believed to be out there waiting to be discovered. The struggle seems to have resulted in competing and perhaps in some instances incompatible theoretical perspectives, which together with often unarticulated, perhaps even unarticulable, knowledge claims leaves nursing unsure of its place in the academy. This reductionist approach has recently been tempered by an apparent general acceptance that a grand theory of nursing might not emerge and might not even be necessary.

The question of what sort of thing nursing is, is not a trivial matter for any predominant vision of nursing will have effects not only on how others perceive it but also on the basis on which nursing practice is predicated. The question may have more immediate importance for academics than it does for practitioners but in time any prevailing view of the nature of nursing (whether this is articulated or not) will influence many aspects of both nursing practice and the way in which nursing practice is organised. It will also have considerable influence on the educational philosophy of those in whose hands the education of students and practitioners of nursing rests.

There are those who seem to accept the idea of 'nursing science' as unproblematic, and the term appears in the title of many university departments, particularly in the USA and in continental Europe, and it appears often in the international nursing literature. As a consequence one might be forgiven for thinking that the idea that nursing is a science, or that there is such a thing as nursing science, has gained a universal acceptance but this is far from the case. There remain many who question the status of nursing as a science and for whom the term 'nursing science' fails to capture the essence of the activity called nursing. In the UK in particular there is scepticism about the possibility of nursing as a science.

The recent emphasis on 'research-based practice' in medicine has led to a similar move in nursing (and elsewhere) and the idea of 'evidence-based practice' is now reflected in nursing curricula. While the idea of 'evidence' rather than 'research' as a basis for nursing practice has gained a foothold in the collective imagination of nurses this is at the cost of definitional imprecision. It enables both those who consider nursing as a science and those who do not the possibility of claiming their own versions of what counts as legitimate evidence. I will return to this point in Chapter 5 but for now it is useful merely to note that those who consider nursing a science tend to take the idea of evidence to mean evidence gained from (positivist) science.

Edwards points out that 'The claim that nursing is a science is a 'class inclusion' claim' (Edwards 2001, p.137). This is to say that before a claim that nursing is a science can be evaluated it is necessary for the characteristics of science to be articulated. However, defining science turns out to be a task not all that much simpler than the task of defining nursing; there remain unresolved debates within the philosophy of science about the true nature of science. Nevertheless, and for the purposes of this account, the view that science is 'a descriptive enterprise' (p.138) will be accepted as this corresponds with the generally accepted understanding of what science is. Science on this account sets out to describe phenomena and this is consistent with science as it appears in the UK school curriculum. As an example, one Key Stage 3 science textbook (Hudson 1998) is divided into three sections entitled: 1) life processes and living things; 2) materials and their properties, and 3) physical properties. These three sections correspond with biology, chemistry and physics respectively (often collectively known as the natural sciences) and the book does indeed attempt to describe the natural world. On this account the claim that nursing is a science is set to fail as nursing is not primarily concerned with describing phenomena. Nursing as a practical activity with normative and evaluative ends is to be distinguished from science with its general aim of description (Edwards 2001).

One response to this failure might be that the description above is unnecessarily focused on the natural sciences. The traditional view that science comprises these three natural sciences effectively prevents the inclusion of any other discipline into the class of science. However the general perception of science as biology, chemistry and physics fails to account for the status of other disciplines that have become known as sciences in their own right. The fact that these other disciplines are known collectively as the social sciences (and hence are to be differentiated from the natural sciences) does not detract from the perceived legitimacy of their claim to be part of that class of disciplines known as the sciences. Psychology and sociology are among the disciplines generally accepted as part of the social sciences. Proponents of nursing as a science might well claim nursing to be a social science.

This claim (that nursing is a social science) is another class inclusion claim and as such requires that we define what is meant by a social science before considering whether or not nursing can be so classified. As with the natural sciences, the social sciences have description as a primary purpose. This helps to explain the general acceptance of psychology and sociology as sciences. In describing the social, rather than the natural, world the social sciences have a more difficult task. There may be no counterpart in the social sciences for what in the natural sciences are termed the laws of nature. Nevertheless, it is the descriptive nature of the social sciences that provides legitimacy for their position as sciences. On this account nursing would once again fail to be a candidate for inclusion as a science and for the same reason. Nursing has normative and evaluative ends whereas the primary task of the social sciences is to describe the social world.

A further response to this failure might be to say that the portrayal of science as primarily descriptive activity is to accept an impoverished view of science. It is a view that is too narrow because part of what we understand science to be includes the practical applications of the results of science. This is to say that while biology, chemistry, physics, psychology and sociology might be considered as pure sciences they form the basis of a range of activities that are known as applied sciences. While it is true that there are some very specific examples of discipline specific applications of the findings of science it is not clear that any one example of what is termed an applied science is a science as such. The difference between an activity that claims to be an applied science and one that merely makes instrumental use of scientific knowledge is unclear which makes any claim that nursing is an applied science difficult to evaluate. Edwards takes the view that:

> If in saying nursing is an applied science it is meant that the findings of science are instigated in a scientific manner…then perhaps nursing is an applied science such as civil engineering… But a crucial difference remains. Nursing actions are answerable to subjective considerations in a way in which applied sciences are not. The fact of whether or not a bridge is a good bridge can be determined by objective criteria… The question of whether or not a pattern of nursing interventions is a good one cannot be determined wholly by objective criteria. (Edwards 2001, p.140)

If nursing is an applied science (understood in the sense of making use of the findings of science) then presumably the practice of nursing is to be based on scientific evidence. And if science is taken to be descriptive activity then this will not only affect the types of evidence that are accepted as legitimate but will also determine the types of questions asked. Opponents of nursing as a science suggest that this is already happening and point to the dominance of certain sorts of evidence which has the effect of restricting the types of questions that can be answered to those that suit quantitative approaches to enquiry. What this approach fails to consider, it is claimed, is the human dimension of nursing activity.

There is, of course, a place for quantitative enquiry, particularly in the technical aspects of nursing, but even where evidence from quantitative enquiry is useful it does not of itself necessarily provide a sufficient basis for practice decisions. When caring for a patient with a wound it is indeed necessary to draw upon the best available scientific evidence but the quantitative evidence that wound type x is best treated using product type z should not be the only evidence a nurse uses to make a final decision regarding the choice of dressing to be applied for in any one given situation. Apart from the fact that the nurse may need to choose between different commercial versions of product type z (versions that may have only subtle and therapeutically insignificant differences) there will be individual differences for in any given patient of which the nurse must take account. Add to this the personal preferences of both patient and nurse together with the nurse's experiences of using different products then it becomes apparent that the choice of dressing rests on more than merely the best available scientific evidence. The need for judgement in weighing up the evidence for the suitability of product z for a patient with wound type x remains precisely because of those individual and contextual factors in the light of which a nurse views a particular patient.

The best dressing for wound type x may well be product type z but if this requires to be redressed every eight hours then its use will only be suitable for patients for whom the dressing can be performed three times each day. A patient in hospital might well meet this criterion but product type z is unlikely to be a good choice for a patient returning home and for whom a daily visit from a community nurse is the best that can be anticipated, or for a homeless person whose contact with a nurse is likely to be no more frequent than once a week. Other factors, such as the nutritional status of the patient and patient acceptability of the product, need to be considered by the nurse and while protocols may exist to provide some guidance the final choice of dressing relies on the professional judgement of the nurse. The nurse who only ever uses scientific evidence (because she or he holds nursing to be a science) and always chooses product type z whenever she or he comes across a patient with wound type x regardless of all other considerations would surely earn our censure for failing to exercise sufficient professional judgement. This is to say, she or he would have displayed a lack of *professional phronesis* for it is necessary that judgements be made in light of a range of available evidence, only some of which will be scientific. So while the use of evidence to guide practice is important it would be an impoverished view of nursing to suggest that the evidence on which practice is based be restricted to scientific evidence alone. Further, while it may be true that nursing makes use of science this, of itself, is not sufficient to classify nursing as a science.

Nursing as a practice

Thus far I have attempted to demonstrate that, despite its seeming prominence, the idea of nursing as a science is contentious at best. I have suggested that there is some benefit in understanding nursing as a practice in the technical sense that MacIntyre uses that term and I will now expand upon this idea. In order to locate this claim within the context of this book it may be helpful to summarise the key components of the argument thus far. I have argued that the recipients of nursing services are *more-than-ordinarily* vulnerable and because of this, the human flourishing of *more-than-ordinarily* vulnerable persons is a legitimate aim of nursing. I have also argued that the existing seemingly dominant view of nursing as a science offers only impoverished account of the nature of nursing.

Bishop and Scudder (1991) reach similar conclusions and distinguish between nursing as a discipline (that is, nursing as a subject of scientific study) and nursing as a practice (that is, the practice of nursing) as a way of avoiding the 'Is nursing a science?' debate.

Drawing from the hermeneutic philosophy of Gadamer, Bishop and Scudder note that practices '...attempt to bring about good in the world' (1991, p.32) and they contrast this with technologies (that is, applied sciences) which have the potential to be used for good or evil.

For Bishop and Scudder this is the reason why it is inappropriate to classify nursing as an applied science. The good that nursing seeks is the well-being of individual patients, which characterises nursing as a moral enterprise with associated moral obligations on the part of individual nurses to provide excellent care. Nursing is thus a caring practice that aims at the good of those who find themselves in receipt of nursing. However, as Edwards notes, 'this is a plausible claim, although not one which distinguishes nursing from other "caring practices" such as parenting, social work and so on' (Edwards 2001, p.164).

In their outline of nursing as a practice Bishop and Scudder do acknowledge the contribution of MacIntyre as well as Gadamer to their thinking both about the nature of a practice in general and about nursing as a practice in particular. They suggest that in MacIntyre's terms nursing can make a legitimate claim to be a practice. Others including Sellman (2000, 2010), Wainwright (1997) and Edwards (2001) have also claimed that nursing is a practice in the MacIntyrean sense.

The claim that will now come under scrutiny is made precisely because the dominant accounts of nursing do not sufficiently capture the essence of the sort of thing that nursing is. As a result I will claim here not only that nursing is a practice but also that nursing can only be properly understood as a practice. I have argued elsewhere (Sellman 2000, 2010) that the features MacIntyre identifies as constitutive of a practice are features recognisable within nursing. I have suggested that the motivation for many who wish to become nurses is explained in a desire to be of help to others; an altruism which has been characterised as an appropriate disposition for nursing. Typically, when asked the question 'Why do you want to be a nurse?' as part of an admissions interview for a pre-registration nursing course, many prospective students will answer to the effect 'Because I want to help people.' Anecdotal as this may be it is the common experience of nursing admissions tutors (at least in the UK) and points to a not unreasonable view that students of nursing are not (at least not in the first instance) primarily interested in external rewards. The external rewards that nursing offers are, generally speaking, easier to acquire elsewhere or in other ways.

While there are historical exceptions to this generalisation (for example, the influx of men into psychiatric nursing in the UK during periods of high unemployment in the first half of the twentieth century) it remains the case that nursing is not easy work and the general perception of nurses themselves is that external rewards of a similar value can be obtained from employment in much less demanding occupations. So while the exact nature of the internal rewards might not be clear to prospective students it is, nevertheless, reasonable to suppose that most prospective candidates recognise that there are internal rewards to be gained from becoming a nurse, even if that initial recognition is limited to an idea that there is some personal satisfaction to be obtained as a nurse.

It is also reasonable to suggest that other internal rewards become important for those who can be identified as good nurses and that these internal rewards become apparent to the student as she or he moves from mere performance of task to purposeful and goal-oriented action in the giving of care; the equivalent in MacIntyre's terms of progression from the inexpert placing of pawns, knights, queens, bishops and so on around the chess board to an appreciation of the skilful and purposeful positioning of particular chess pieces with a specific goal or set of goals in mind. The later stages of both represent a certain level of perspicacity together with an engagement with an activity not merely as an activity but as a practice in this MacIntyrean sense.

Of course, as Edwards points out, nursing could be both a science and a practice, for it is clear that MacIntyre understands science (conducted properly) as a practice. Thus the rejection of nursing as a science is not a necessary phase in coming to view nursing as a practice. Nevertheless, a critical review of the claim that nursing is a science is necessary if we are to take seriously any attempt to classify the activity of nursing. There may be other, more plausible, class inclusion claims for nursing but one advantage of regarding nursing as a practice is that such possibilities are not excluded; in other words, it is a position which allows for other conceptions of nursing without invalidating the idea of nursing being a practice as well as belonging some other class of things. All I have done here is to conclude, as others (notably, Bishop and Scudder 1991 and Edwards 2001) have done that the conception of nursing as a science is, at best, a fragile idea.

We can now return to MacIntyre's outline of a practice as:

> any coherent and complex form of socially established cooperative human activity through which goods internal to that form of activity are realized in the course of trying to achieve those standards of excellence which are appropriate to, and partially definitive of, that form of activity, with the result that human

powers to achieve excellence, and human conceptions of ends and goods involved are systematically extended. (MacIntyre 1985, p.187)

and assess the extent to which nursing fits this description. Certainly we can point to nursing as a 'socially established cooperative activity' so we can say that the first criterion is met. Of greater difficulty is how far it is correct to say that there are goods internal to nursing that are constitutive of nursing. The answer to this question would seem to be predetermined by whatever understanding of nursing is taken as given. To take a view that nursing is no more than as a series of tasks to be completed is to understand nursing as a mere technical activity no different from any other form of work in which that work is solely a means of obtaining the external good of money. From such a position it would be strange to imagine nursing as a practice – so it seems that those with this view are unable to conceive of nursing as a practice unless they can be persuaded that there is more to it than this instrumental view suggests. Apart from those who value the goods of effectiveness more that the goods of excellence, most individuals would understand that good nursing is not described by such an impoverished account. Of course, good nursing requires the acquisition of competency in whichever set of necessary skills are required for nursing as practised in any particular situation but as intimated earlier (and as will be discussed later) even the safe and efficient accomplishment of a set of skills does not make a good nurse unless a good nurse is understood as a mere technician.

If it is correct to say that nursing is concerned with the flourishing of *more-than-ordinarily* vulnerable persons then this professional ideal of service (as Sockett calls it) is important in terms of both process and outcome. This is to say, that human flourishing is valued as both ends and means of practice because human flourishing by definition requires attention to the general effects on well-being, not just on, for example, the physical results of interventions. In addition, the pursuit of whichever excellences are appropriate to a practice is a necessary component of that practice. The excellences of nursing as a practice include the provision of a high standard of nursing care however this is defined within any particular interaction between nurse(s) and patient(s). The internal goods associated with the pursuit of this ideal might include the professional satisfaction of a job well done and pleasure at the attempt of making a positive difference to the well-being of a patient. As MacIntyre notes, in a practice the achievement of such internal goods requires their pursuit to be consistent with (at a minimum) the core virtues of honesty, courage and justice. As such, engaging with a practice not only provides a place in modernity for virtues to flourish but also offers a route by which the virtues can be encouraged as a result of habituation and as a result of the recognition by practitioners that the goods internal to that practice are only available if one engages with the activity as a practice. Thus it would seem that nursing does indeed meet the second criterion insofar as nursing can be said to offer the possibility of realising goods internal to nursing practice. Further, it seems that the pursuit of excellence in the practice of nursing is a reality for those nurses who take seriously the business of nursing; that is, as the pursuit of the professional ideal of service for the betterment of patients. Thus, in pursuit of nursing as a practice not only is the flourishing of patients facilitated but also the flourishing of nurses *qua* humans is enabled.

The core virtues of practices

The virtues of honesty, courage and justice are of central importance to a practice precisely because they offer a defence against the corrupting influences of institutions and the associated tendency of emphases on goods of effectiveness. Without these three virtues the essential connection between ends and means is lost; in other words, practices cannot survive without the virtues of honesty, courage and justice. MacIntyre provides an outline sketch of the central importance of these three virtues in *After Virtue*. He says of a practice:

> its [internal] goods can only be achieved by subordinating ourselves within the practice in our relationship to other practitioners. We have to learn to recognize what is due to whom; we have to be prepared to take whatever self-endangering risks are demanded along the way; and we have to listen carefully to what we are told about our own inadequacies and to reply with the same carefulness for the facts. In other words we have to accept as necessary components of any practice with internal goods and standards of excellence the virtues of justice, courage and honesty. (MacIntyre 1985, p.191)

In the brief discussion that follows these words MacIntyre notes that dishonesty between those engaged in a practice jeopardises relationships between practitioners in terms of the pursuit of the communal goods of that practice. Similarly, a failure of justice or of courage damages the relationships between those engaged in the practice and renders the pursuit of the internal goods meaningless. For, as he points out, the pursuit of internal goods is not competitive in the way that the pursuit of external goods often is. Pursuit of the prize money for winning a major chess championship inevitably requires that one person's success is everybody else's failure, whereas the internal goods of a practice are freely available to all those who engage with it as a practice. Any competition that exists within practices is generally aimed at the pursuit of excellence within that practice and as well as being of benefit for the individual, this is of benefit for the community of practitioners and beyond. In the case of nursing, the benefit extends to individual patients as well as to the health and welfare of the general community.

If nursing is a practice then the virtues of honesty, justice and courage are of central importance and the cultivation of these three virtues is an essential part of what nurses engaged with nursing as a practice must pursue. The idea that nurses should be honest and just is consistent both with general assumptions of how nurses should behave and with professional expectations. However, the idea that nurses should be courageous is not so obvious although it should take only a moment of reflection to recognise that in those situations where the best interests of patients might be at risk the requirement for nurses to stand up and be counted (as it were) may require a great deal of courage; whistleblowers, for example, are often subject to considerable professional and personal costs for their efforts.

While the words used in nursing codes in different nation states may vary, MacIntyre's primary virtues of honesty, justice and courage are invariably present. If nursing codes are attempts to articulate the core values of the profession then the consistency over time of the expression of MacIntyre's core virtues adds weight to the contention that nursing is a practice. And, as noted in the introduction to this book, professional codes are revised periodically, which means that to quote directly from any one particular nursing code is to anticipate that the quote may quickly become out of date. Nevertheless, and for the purposes of illustration, I will quote from the Canadian nurses' code current at the time of writing. And I am confident that the reader will find these same entreaties to act expressed in their own current code.

The injunction to be honest is clearly articulated:

> Nurses recognize, respect and promote a person's right to be informed and make decisions. (CNA 2008, p.11)

> Nurses do not engage in any form of lying…they refuse to be complicit in such behaviours. (p.17)

> Nurses are honest… (p.18)

The injunction to be just is similarly unequivocal:

> When providing care, nurses do not discriminate on the basis of a person's race, ethnicity, culture, political and spiritual beliefs, social or marital status, gender, sexual orientation, age, health status, place of origin, lifestyle, mental or physical ability or socio-economic status or any other attribute. (CNA 2008, p.17)

> Nurses make fair decisions about the allocation of resources under their control based on the needs of persons, groups or communities for whom they are providing care. (p.17)

The injunction to be courageous is less explicit but can be found in such statements as:

> Nurses question and intervene to address unsafe, non-compassionate, unethical or incompetent practice or condition that interfere with their ability to provide safe, compassionate, competent care. (CNA 2008, p.9)

This last quote seems to require a nurse to exhibit considerable courage, particularly in those circumstances where a failure to act would be to fail to practise in ways consistent with those injunctions.

Being professionally accountable for one's acts and omissions can take a great deal of courage when faced with instructions from managers or more senior health care professionals to act in ways inconsistent with the professional ideal of service. Indeed, acting in ways consistent with the types of injunctions expressed in the codes requires courage in the face of competing demands: being truthful to patients when more senior staff demand the withholding of some pertinent information from a client is difficult in the traditional hierarchy of health care; ensuring that a homeless person or a 'drunk' gets the care they need when there is a general view that such patients are not worth bothering with or are a waste of time or resources requires considerable self-assurance; and refusal to undertake a task for which one is not competent when asked to do so by a more senior professional who says she or he will take responsibility can make a nurse unpopular and result in a reputation of being 'difficult'. Following the injunctions of nursing codes in these sorts of circumstances (which are not unusual) requires a great deal of courage. Without courage nurses will be tempted to 'give in' to these pressures: the desire to conform to local norms and to be accepted, the need to get a good grade or reference, and the wish not to have to battle everyday at work can all weaken the will to practise in ways consistent with the code. As a result practice can insidiously creep away from the ideal to the detriment of the care and protection of *more-than-ordinarily* vulnerable persons. Those who have, or who aim for, the virtues of honesty, justice and courage will be better able to recognise corrupting influences and better able to act in honest, just and courageous ways. It seems we have good reason for asking nurses to cultivate the virtues because such nurses are better able to withstand pressures that might otherwise corrupt.

As I suggested earlier in this chapter, the virtues of honesty, justice and courage are relatively uncontentious and, as noted above, those nurses who are disposed to act in cohort with these virtues will be in a relatively strong position to resist practice-corrupting influences. Honesty, justice and courage are centrally important in the practice of nursing but there are other necessary dispositions. In Chapters 4 and 5 I offer an account of trustworthiness and open-mindedness respectively and I provide an outline of the important place these two particular dispositions have in the practice of nursing.

4 Trust and Trustworthiness

As suggested at the end of Chapter 3, trust is generally considered an important aspect of nursing. Generally speaking, it is expected that patients should be able to trust nurses (as well as other health and social care practitioners) and the importance of this idea is given formal expression in nursing codes (for example, ANA 2001; CNA 2008; NMC 2008). Given this emphasis, it might come as a surprise to find that the nursing literature on trust and trustworthiness is sparse. This suggests a general view that issues of trust and trustworthiness are unproblematic.

However, in such literature on trust and trustworthiness as exists, there are some who believe otherwise. It may be that rather than being suggestive of being uncontentious or unproblematic, the paucity of literature reflects a general failure to recognise problems associated with being trustworthy, particularly in professional life – although Banks and Gallagher (2009) do begin to outline some of the difficulties associated with trust in the professional life of nurses and social workers. Additionally, and despite its significance for the moral life of persons, trust has received relatively scant attention from philosophers in general and from moral philosophers in particular. As Baier (1986) points out, one feature of existing accounts is the tendency to dwell almost exclusively on trust as something that occurs between rational adults. This failure of perspective limits discussions of trust for the most part to relationships between competent adults. On these accounts individuals whose rational capacities are compromised or diminished, or who are otherwise unable to express their autonomy, would appear to be excluded. The conceptions of trust that claim trust is solely a matter of contractual agreement(s) between equally autonomous adults will struggle to account for some aspects of everyday experiences of trust, particularly within health care situations. Trust invariably involves persons at different times and in different ways throughout their lives and involves them, moreover, when they are sometimes more and sometimes less autonomous, sometimes more and sometimes less dependent, sometimes more and sometimes less powerful, and sometimes more and sometimes less vulnerable.

Everyday understandings of trust can account for these variations in capacities in ways that some philosophical, sociological and psychological accounts cannot. Attempts to clarify the nature of trust have led to a series of distinctions between different forms of trust as well as between trust on the one hand and reliance, confidence, faith, hope and belief on the other. These distinctions are undoubtedly helpful in providing clarity, for trust is indeed different from confidence, faith, hope and belief, but this approach can lead the unwary into a pedantic cul-de-sac. Nevertheless, each has its place in aiding our understanding of trust. There is little doubt that confusion between different meanings of trust can easily arise, especially when (overly) simplistic distinctions are made. Thus the first task of this chapter is to consider the nature of trust.

Once we have a conception of trust sufficiently able to account for both variations in the capacities of individuals and for the relative differences in power between them that this inevitably entails, it should be possible to begin the task of identifying the place of trust and trustworthiness in caring for *more-than-ordinarily* vulnerable persons. Annette Baier reminds us of the intimate connection between trust and vulnerability when she states: 'Trust...on...first approximation, is accepted vulnerability to another's possible but not expected ill will (or lack of goodwill) toward one' (Baier 1986, p.235). On this view it is when we place trust that we expose, or at least acknowledge, our vulnerability,[11] but this is to recognise only one aspect of the complex relationship between trust and vulnerability. For it is equally true to say, as I have implied in my earlier discussion, that it is because we are vulnerable that we must place trust; and it is when we are *more-than-ordinarily* vulnerable that our need to trust is at its most pressing. The received wisdom is (at least since the time of Florence Nightingale) that a nurse should be trustworthy. Yet, as with other assumed 'qualities' that nurses are supposed to exhibit, not only are the reasons why a nurse ought to be trustworthy somewhat obscure, but also the nature and the expression of this trustworthiness is largely unstable. Thus the second task of this chapter is to consider the place of trust and trustworthiness in the practice of nursing. Nancy Potter (2002) argues for trustworthiness as a virtue and tempting as this is, it is far from clear that it can be considered a virtue as such for reasons that will be rehearsed as the chapter progresses. I will claim that while it may not be a virtue there is a logic in understanding trustworthiness as a professional virtue in the sense that I have defined that term in Chapter 1.

Background trust

Background trust is generally taken to be important for without it, it would be difficult to sustain any sense of well-being or security in everyday life. Bernard Williams (2002) makes the observation that there remains a background of trust in all but the most extreme situations. This background of trust is what allows us to make sense of our social relationships. It makes possible the idea that, for the most part, as Baier (1986) suggests, others neither intend us harm nor intend to interfere unnecessarily with us as we live out our lives. Without this general sense of background trust it is difficult to imagine how human flourishing could occur. At those times and in those places where people have reason to experience a high level of background *distrust* there is likely to be an air of disquiet, suspicion and anxiety. Such things are surely obstacles to human flourishing. However, as with other forms of trust, background trust can be compromised and once lost, may be difficult to re-establish. This fragility of trust is well documented. In our own time, the events of September 11, 2001 have given us reason to be wary of being complacent about the components of our general background trust. Of course, the Stoics would want to warn us against any sort of complacency in an idea of general background trust precisely because it increases our vulnerability. And while we do well to heed this warning, it remains the case that a background of trust appears to be necessary for human flourishing. Much might be said about background trust but for the purposes of the present discussion it is sufficient to recognise that its existence enables other forms of trust to flourish.

For present purposes it is necessary to come to an understanding of the nature of some of these others forms of trust because it is from a knowledge of trust that we can begin to understand what it is to be trustworthy. And once we have identified the features of trustworthiness we can set about, with some confidence, the further task of exploring ways in which to foster learning environments conducive to the development of the professional virtue of trustworthiness. This of course presupposes that trust and trustworthiness are important for nursing, and in due course I will argue that being trustworthy contributes to the human flourishing of those in receipt of nursing care; that is, contributes towards the flourishing of *more-than-ordinarily* vulnerable persons.

The nature of trust

The literature on trust is dominated by accounts located primarily in either the discipline of psychology or the discipline of sociology, both of which lay claim to the phenomenon. Central to the various claims of psychology is the idea that trust is an attitude of mind, a feature of the psyche, an attribute of an individual nature; whereas sociological descriptions tend to emphasise trust as some form of social contract. By and large, both disciplines assume trust involves competent adults able to engage as equal contributors to the construction of, respectively, individual or social relationships. In addition, there is a literature in philosophy some of which begins to recognise the significance of the power differentials between individuals in many trust relationships. Where trust is a matter for discussion in the nursing literature these discussions tend to demonstrate allegiance to either psychological or sociological traditions.

Typically those who enter the debate on the nature of trust become embroiled in attempts to distance the idea of trust from the ideas of, for example, hope, faith, confidence, belief and reliance. Yet defining trust invariably requires the use of those same terms. This suggests inter alia that the nature of trust is such as to make the disaggregation project difficult. This is not to say that the attempts are futile, for discussion provides a reminder of the important issues within matters of trust and the related ideas of hope, faith, confidence, belief and reliance. So while it is a requirement for Baier that trust involves the belief that others have a good will towards one (and for her this is what distinguishes it from mere reliance), O'Neill notes that we 'Sometimes…know that good will is lacking, and yet we trust' (O'Neill 2002, p.14), illustrating the point by noting that 'A patient may know a doctor finds him

WHAT MAKES A GOOD NURSE

particularly irritating and bears him little good will, and yet trust the doctor to exercise proper professional judgement' (p.14). It is not clear whether what O'Neill describes here is trust or reliance. The patient might not believe the doctor has a good will towards him but may still trust the doctor to act professionally (what Seligman (1997) describes as 'systems trust'). Alternatively the patient may not trust the doctor in any sense but merely rely on him because there is no other choice – in this respect reliance begins to look rather like hope. Presumably, Baier would say that O'Neill's example is simply a case of reliance; that the patient is unable to trust and therefore has no choice but to rely upon the doctor's professionalism, or (in O'Neill's terms) upon systems of accountability set up to ensure patients are treated fairly regardless of the personal feelings of physicians. Thus what we can recognise in these disagreements is not necessarily disagreement about the essence of trust, but rather disagreement about distinctions between trust and reliance.

Trust as part of a family of ideas

One thing we might take from this is the idea that trust is part of a family of ideas; a family that includes belief, hope, faith, confidence and reliance. Each can be distinguished from trust but in some instances it can be hard to tell them apart, although, following Baier, it will be allowed that it is the assumption of good will towards us that makes the difference, at least insofar as we focus on differences between trust and confidence/reliance (the defence of good will as the essential feature of trust is threaded throughout the remainder of this section of the current chapter). Baier's example that we may 'trust our enemies not to fire at us when we lay down our arms and put out a white flag' (1986, p.234) has been criticised for assuming a motivation of good will (or at least a lack of an ill will) on the part of our enemy. Holton (1994) notes that when we surrender our enemy may refrain from shooting us not from good will, but from a sense of duty towards prisoners, or because that is what he is trained to do as a soldier. He may actually have a desire to do us harm especially if he blames us as the enemy who has caused him suffering, loss of loved ones and so on. So while we might say that we trust him not to shoot us as we surrender, we might also say that we hope, or we believe, or have faith, or have confidence, that our enemy will conform to the practice of refraining from harming those who have surrendered. We might infer any of these because at the time of surrendering we do not know his motivation. But to follow this approach is to misconstrue the nature of trust, for this would be to conclude that we can only give trust when we are certain that the other has good will towards us. But this cannot be right for trust is only an issue in matters of uncertainty. We cannot know that those in whom we place our trust have good will towards us – if we could be sure about this it would no longer be a matter of trust. It is only because we cannot be sure about others' good will towards us that we must consider whether or not to trust and sometimes our trust will turn out to have been misplaced. Thus we trust when we believe that those in whom we are prepared to trust have a good will toward us. And this belief in others' good will is what distinguishes trust from the other ideas in the trust family of ideas.

Hart comes close to suggesting a family of ideas around trust when he suggests:

> a continuum of words connoting *belief* based on the degree on which they rest on evidence of the senses. Faith requires no evidence; trust is an expectation based on inconclusive evidence, is tolerant of uncertainty or risk; confidence is a strong conviction based on substantial evidence or logical deduction. (Hart 1988, p.187; original emphasis)

So for Hart trust lies between, and can be distinguished from, both faith and confidence. He further suggests that reliance represents 'complete confidence' (p.187): a state in which belief is no longer necessary, or rather, where the evidence equates to full knowledge and certainty. Others (including Baier) use reliance in the sense (more or less) that Hart uses confidence; so to rely on someone to do a thing is to have confidence that they will do it. While there may remain some subtle differences between reliance and confidence the two terms will be used throughout this chapter in the way I have outlined above. Hart's is a useful, if non-specific, metric that allows us to recognise that there are distinctions to be made between trust and faith on the one hand, and trust and confidence on the other on the basis of the evidence available to us.

Hart's approach does have the advantage of retaining some aspects of everyday understandings of three inter-related terms (and the associated ideas) even if it does not provide us with a way of determining between marginal cases. However, if we accept the idea that there is a certain dynamic in the use of these terms and that efforts to define any of them too rigidly may be to confine meaning unnecessarily (at least for present purposes) then we can proceed with the task in hand. That task is to establish a working construct of trust that accounts for differences in power of agents in trust relationships between patients and professionals (specifically nurses) within health and social care environments. To begin this task we must now turn to a defence of Baier's conception of trust.

Trust and good will

For Baier (1986) trust is a particular form of reliance (or confidence in Hart's terms), that is, a reliance on the good will (or at least the absence of ill will) of others. This distinction is common in discussions on the nature of trust although it is not a distinction without difficulties. Holton rejects the requirement for good will on two grounds: 'In the first place...the confidence trickster might rely on your goodwill without trusting you. Secondly...I can trust a person without relying on their goodwill towards me' (Holton 1994, p.65); the latter reflects the criticism made by O'Neill discussed briefly earlier.

In the first example Holton confuses the good will of the one trusting with the good will of the one being trusted. Certainly it is true that the confidence trickster may rely on his victims' good will, that is after all part of the nature of 'the con', but as Baier notes it is confidence tricksters, amongst others, who understand the essential features of trust and use them for instrumental purposes. That the confidence trickster uses the good will of others in exploitative ways may illustrate a problem of principle (that is, it may demonstrate a need for a guiding principle to help us avoid falling victim to the abuse of our trust) but it does not of itself render Baier's definition redundant. In fact it provides support to the idea that good will is an essential feature of trust, for what Holton neglects in this example is the trust shown by the victim. The only thing the victim is guilty of is a misplaced trust; a trust based on the belief that the other has a good will toward her. The pretence of trustworthiness merely serves to illustrate the confidence trickster's ability to use the features of trust, and of trustworthiness, as means for his own instrumental ends.

TRUST AND TRUSTWORTHINESS

To illustrate his second objection Holton notes that a divorced parent may not have good will toward her ex-partner but may well trust him with their children. But Holton appears to have fallen into a narrow view of Baier's conception of the relationship between trust and good will. For Baier, it is a good will toward whatever it is that we value when we are thinking about placing trust in another. To trust one's ex-partner to care for the children is to place trust in her or his good will towards the children rather than towards one's self. If there is sufficient doubt about the ex-partner's good will toward the children then we might be forced to rely on them to care for the children but this would not be a matter of trust. This example points to the issue of the context in which trust occurs. One thing that our everyday understandings of what we mean when we say we trust have in common is the context bound nature of meaning. It is because we understand the context in which the term trust is used that we can, generally speaking, understand who is being trusted with what, as well as what it is that trust requires of us, in different situations.

It seems then that good will is an essential feature of trust for as Potter reminds us 'An attitude of indifference to particular persons does not foster a great degree of trust even if "right actions" are performed' (Potter 2002, p.6). In this respect Potter has enlarged upon Baier's distinction between trust and reliance. In her discussion Potter recognises that there is a 'sort of trust' that accompanies, for example, trusting another not to lie when one knows that she or he holds it as a matter of principle that lying is wrong. But for Potter, this sort of trust is unsatisfactory because it lacks any sense in which the one who can be trusted not to lie needs to have good will towards any one particular person. Indeed, on this account one who is known to have an ill will towards another but can still be trusted not to lie would be exhibiting a Kantian morality; that is, acting against rather than in concert with inclination. I suggest that when we say we trust someone in this way we make a distinction between two different senses of trust. In one sense we trust someone to do a particular thing (so this is a type of instrumental trust for it is a means to some specified end) in the other we trust someone because of the sort of person they are. It might be argued that the type of instrumental trust identified here is not trust at all but reliance – for one can rely on a deontologist not to lie but one might not trust them to care for the goods one holds dear. In either case we might say there is actually a threefold distinction to be made between reliance, and two discrete forms of trust: 1) trust in the context of a particular matter, and 2) full trust.

This discussion points to a role for discretion in matters of trust. We use discretion to differentiate between what we mean when we say we trust a friend and when we say we trust a friend in some specific way or to do a particular thing. We use discretion when we say of someone that we would trust them with our life. And we use discretion when we decide who to trust and in what respect. We know that those in whom we place trust have the potential to harm us but in trusting them we trust that they use their discretion to act in trustworthy ways in respect of the trust we have placed in them. When we trust someone not to lie solely as a matter of principle we recognise an absence of discretion on their part. If a trusted person cannot be trusted to act with the discretion that comes from an understanding of why that which is entrusted to them is of value to the person doing the trusting then it seems we are trusting unwisely. The practical application of this is that we would be well advised to acknowledge the distinction between trust and reliance, especially our tendency (if we have such) to mistake others' allegiance to abstract duty as trustworthiness. If only because while those who do adhere to duty might be reliable in terms of that duty, they cannot be trusted not to override their concern for our individual well-being or flourishing. It is this that leads Potter to conclude that 'In evaluating someone's trustworthiness…we need to know that she can be counted on, as a matter of the sort of person she is, to take care of those things with which we are considering entrusting her' (Potter 2002, p.7). In coming to a view about the trustworthiness of another we are making an assessment of their character; an assessment, that is, of their dispositional stance towards us.

Holton pursues the idea of a 'participant stance' (Holton 1994, p.66) as part of his critique of Baier's account. Baier's claim that it is good will (or a lack of ill will) towards one that turns mere reliance into trust rests upon the recognition that it is when we lose trust that we can see the difference between trust and reliance. She illustrates the point thus: 'We may rely on our fellows' fear of the newly appointed security guards in shops to deter them from injecting poison into the food on the shelves, once we have ceased to trust them' (Baier 1986, p.234). Hotlon again takes Baier to task, claiming that she misconstrues the nature of reliance. Holton suggests that what we rely on in this example is the security guards' ability to prevent unauthorised access to the food rather than, necessarily, the potential poisoner's fear of getting caught. But this seems an unnecessary distraction as both Baier and Holton agree that there is a distinction to be made between trust and reliance. Despite Holton's criticism, Baier's example serves to illustrate the distinction, for her point is that in ceasing to trust we no longer take others' good will (or lack of ill will) toward us to exist. When we trust, it is the intentions of the other towards us that matters: we seek some (re)assurance of their good will; when we merely rely, the motivation of those on whom we now rely becomes irrelevant. So even if, as Holton claims, Baier has misconstrued the nature of reliance in the security guard example it does not matter. We can accept both Holton's and Baier's interpretation without losing sight of the distinction both want to make. To trust and to rely require us to make predictions about the likely future behaviour of others; in the former we make predications based upon our sense of the extent to which the other has a good will (or an absence of ill will) towards us, in the latter we make a prediction based on a recognition that we cannot rely on their good will.

Holton's alternative is the 'participant stance' we adopt: a stance that reflects how we will be towards something or someone. Thus when we rely and are disappointed we may be angry but when our trust is betrayed we feel some personal slight. For Holton it is this stance that determines whether we demonstrate trust or reliance. However his use of the example of our anger when our car breaks down suggests that he has in mind a distinction between reliance on an object and trust in persons or as Luhmann puts it 'Trust remains vital in interpersonal relations, but participation in functional systems…requires confidence' (Luhmann 1988, p.102). There is a certain intuitive logic as well as a sense of the ordinary everyday meaning of trust and its variants in the idea that one places trust in persons but merely relies on objects, but it is, I suspect, an analysis that remains too simplistic. I think Baier would agree that to trust is to adopt a stance, but that stance involves a *belief* that the person in whom one trusts has a good will towards one; and this emphasis on belief in others' good will appears to overcome the objections of both Holton and O'Neill.

Willingness to trust

One thing that emerges from the discussion thus far is the notion of a proper amount of trust, or an appropriate amount of distrust. I have indicated that trust is situated within individuals. What we aim for when we trust (or distrust) is the right amount of trust (or distrust). We sometimes get it wrong: we sometimes trust too much and we sometimes trust too little; we sometimes distrust too much and sometimes distrust too little. Indeed, we might find these failures of trust easier to identify in other people than we do in ourselves for the subjective and individual nature of our trust does not lend itself to rigid definition. So we might say, following Aristotle, that trust (or distrust) is a mean between trusting (or distrusting) too much and trusting (or distrusting) too little. Figure 4.1 provides this in representational form.

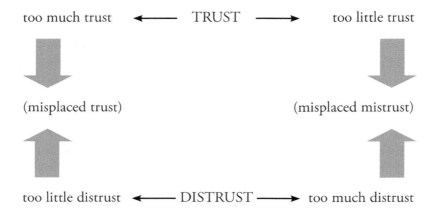

Figure 4.1 Willingness to trust (and distrust) as a mean

Viewed in this way our willingness to trust (or distrust) can be seen as a virtue located at a mean between an excess and a deficiency. It is important to note that the mean is not at a central point, rather it lies between an excess and a deficiency and the precise location is determined by the circumstances in which trust or distrust is called upon. I have borrowed O'Neill's (2002) terms of *misplaced trust* to represent too much trust/too little distrust and *misplaced mistrust* to represent too little trust/too much distrust. Used in this way it might appear unnecessary to distinguish between trust and distrust. But while, for example, too little trust and too much distrust can be collapsed into a single idea there are other distinctions to be made between trust and distrust. There is a tendency to view trust as positive and distrust as negative but this is overly simplistic. As White (1996) points out, an appropriate amount of distrust in institutions is something we should encourage as a positive civic virtue because this has the overall effect of assisting those institutions to be recognised as trustworthy. Similarly, the possibility of pathological trust (that is, a blind trust that can lead to harm and be an obstacle to human flourishing) is something that cannot be considered as positive. Additionally, it is true to say that a willingness to trust appropriately is the primary virtue in personal relationships where distrust would be tend to be destructive.

I noted earlier that we trust unwisely when we trust someone who neither understands the value we put on that which we entrust to them nor has the necessary discretion to recognise the boundaries that a given trust entails. Under normal circumstances, we cannot abrogate responsibility for making judgements about others' trustworthiness when we exercise trust. General everyday experience suggests that, leaving aside the confidence trickster who offers a simulacrum of trustworthiness, most of us approximate the mean of trust (or distrust) more often than not. And learning to aim for the mean (trusting the right amount for a given situation) is important if we are not to be disappointed when we trust. Part of what aiming for the mean entails is recognising in others those things about them that give us confidence in their discretion in looking after whatever it is they have been entrusted with. The discretion of the trusted person to act in ways consistent with the value given by the one who trusts to whatever has been entrusted is crucial to the assessment of the trusted person's trustworthiness (at least from the point of view of the one doing the trusting). So the person who is trusted to look after one's home while one is on vacation and takes it upon her or himself to redecorate is demonstrating a failure of trust by going beyond what is required of trust in that context.[12] Similarly the person who does not do enough to care for that with which she or he has been entrusted is also guilty of a failure of trust *from the perspective of the one doing the trusting*. These examples might be construed as failures of trust on the part of both the one doing the trusting (misplaced trust) and the one being trusted (untrustworthiness). That such interdependency between the trusting and the trusted exists should come as no surprise given the complex nature of human relationships. One set of problems for trust that arises from this insight is the way in which actors in any trust relationship determine the boundaries of discretion in situations when trust is unsought, unrecognised or unwanted. A discussion of this particular and important set of issues for trust lies beyond the scope of this book for here we are concerned with the willingness to trust and its relationship with trusting wisely.

A willingness to trust in the right measure is what Baier refers to as appropriate trust. Appropriate trust requires the use of discretion in the attempt to determine whether or not someone has a good will towards us. It is our assessment of others' good will towards us that enables us to distinguish between each of the ideas of hope, faith, confidence, belief and reliance on the one hand and trust on the other. The essential point here is that the degree of trust any one individual may allow is dependent upon both the importance that individual places upon the trust required for a particular given situation and the individual's assessment of the other's good will toward one. This is to recognise that trust is relative to an individual and has limits determined by particular situations. Thus one may trust, for example, another to do a particular thing, or to act in a particular way; or one may merely trust another to a lesser or greater extent in some respects but not in others. In some cases one may merely trust another, period, although I take this to be a rare phenomenon indeed.

A conception of trust

Baier's emphasis on good will as the defining component of trust is central to the conception of trust accepted for the purposes of this discussion. As such we can say that we trust when we believe that those in whom we place our trust have a good will towards us.

This requirement for belief might be construed as requiring the capacity of independent practical reasoning as discussed in Chapter 3 and under normal circumstances this would be a reasonable requirement. However, as already noted, it is with the flourishing of *more-than-ordinarily* vulnerable persons, many of whom will have a reduced capacity for independent practical reasoning, that this book is primarily concerned and one might be forgiven for assuming that such persons are therefore unable to trust as such. But rather that being a defining attribute of trust, the requirement for belief is relative and contingent insofar as it is a necessary component only as far as it is possible for any given individual to exhibit. Thus for some it will be a matter of a general trust in health care that enables us to say that this or that person trusts when they are unable to make a conscious decision to trust in particular circumstances. The person lying unconscious following a road traffic incident or during a surgical operation fits this description. We can imagine that the former has a general background trust in health care professionals to respond appropriately to a road traffic incident and that the latter has, by virtue of consenting to surgery, expressed a trust in health care professionals to act in her or his best interest while anaesthetised. For others, those whose rational capacities have never developed beyond certain infantile levels, trust may be a reflection of a 'belief' in those on whom the person is dependent, in the sense in which Baier characterises infant trust as the sort of trust needed if an infant is to survive.

Thus here is no necessity for a contract between equally competent persons for it to be said that trust exists between persons. The fact is, that in any trust relationship there is likely to be a power differential although often we may not notice this. When we trust in an institution we are most likely to recognise that we are on the weaker end of the power differential. Similarly when we trust in a person we allow them some power over our affairs. As Baier notes, in allowing others this power over us we allow them to be in a position to harm us and we accept a vulnerability. For those people whose vulnerability is already exposed, to trust in others increases their vulnerability. And yet it is a feature of the human condition that when we are vulnerable we have a greater need to trust others to care for those things we value. If I value my health, and if I find my ability to care for my health is compromised I need the help of others, and it would seem preferable to trust rather than merely rely upon those others.

The place of trust in nursing practice

We trust, then, *when we believe* those in whom we are placing our trust are worthy of that trust; that is when we believe them to be trustworthy. In Baier's example, we trust our enemy not to shoot us as we surrender *when we believe* that he has a good will toward us. Thus our assessment of the trustworthiness of others is a matter of some importance, and in assessing that trustworthiness we are making a judgement about their good will toward us. On this account those who claim to be trustworthy, as nurses often do, must not only have a good will towards patients but must also be seen to have a good will. For it is when we believe that another has a good will towards us that we can say we trust, rather than, say, merely hope or rely.

That patients should trust nurses and that nurses should be trustworthy are two ideas generally held to be important in the practice of nursing. But why should this be so? Why is trust important here? Surely all that is needed is that patients have confidence in the systems of regulation for practising nurses? If patients can rely on the competence of nurses why is there a need for anything else? The reassurance these things provide allows one to know that when one becomes a patient one is in safe hands. Why isn't this enough? If trust and trustworthiness are so important, what is it that they add?

Given that the enterprise of health and social care is generally focused on helping individuals to maximise their potential for health (broadly defined) and given that nursing practice requires interactions between nurses and patients, and that this inevitably gives rise to (inter)personal relationships, then it is not unreasonable to locate the discussion (at least in the first instance) in terms of personal trust. But first it is necessary to take a brief historical view of the story of trust in health care.

The tradition of trust in health care

As with many aspects of nursing, the roots of the tradition of trust are to be found in medicine. The necessity of trust for medical practice is articulated in the Hippocratic Oath and, despite challenges to medical and professional domination of health care provision, this remains a powerful influence on the view that patients should place their trust in doctors and other health care professionals. Carlton sums this up when she says: 'Physicians believe that patients have an obligation to accept their recommendations for treatment... Patients *must* trust their physicians as a condition of the therapeutic enterprise' (Carlton 1978, p.24; emphasis added). What this tradition requires is that doctors and, by extension, other health care professionals (including nurses) act in the best interests of patients, and this is part of what seems to be meant by trust in professional–patient relationships. Quite what acting in a patient's best interests actually involves, and therefore what it is that health care professionals can be trusted with or to do changes over time and remains a matter of debate, not only within and between health care professionals but also between health care professionals on the one hand and patients and the general public on the other. Medicine (at least in the UK) remains an inherently conservative profession with entrenched hierarchical power relationships that tend to militate against reform. For example, medicine, in the form of the British Medical Association, has a history of holding out against changes including objections to the creation of the NHS and, more recently, to proposed changes both to the consultant contract and to junior doctors' working hours. In medical practice this intrinsic conservatism leads in some cases to the continuance of discredited practices in the face of both evidence of the need for reform and of a demand for change.

In assumptions about what it means to be entrusted with the health of patients doctors (and other health care professionals) have often taken it upon themselves to make decisions affecting individuals without reference to individual patients' own perspectives of the limits of discretion involved in allowing such trust. Thus, for example, generalised practices such as withholding information from dying patients about the fact of their dying may have been justifiable when medicine had little to offer beyond identifying the terminal stage of a life. But medicine's inherent conservatism has allowed this practice of 'benevolent paternalism' to continue in the form of therapeutic privilege (by which a doctor can use discretion to withhold information she or he considers to be harmful to the health of the patient) and in the concession given to doctors in the UK Data Protection Act whereby the right of access to medical information is only partial insofar as a medical practitioner retains the right, when a patient requests to see her or his medical records, to remove information that the doctor believes not in the patient's best interest to read. While such clauses may well emerge from good intentions, it is clear that restrictions of this type offer those with a tendency not to trust the medical establishment further reason to be suspicious of health care practitioners. This can, therefore, contribute to a climate of distrust *from the patients' perspective*. Indeed, the cynic would have some justification in noting that leaving this gate-keeping function in the hands of the same professionals who stand to be criticised provides the very conditions in which corruption and untrustworthiness can thrive. All this serves to reinforce the dispositions of those who are disinclined to trust health care professionals.

Until the breakaway from the direct and overt domination of medicine (a process that began in the UK during the 1960s and culminated with the publication of the first UK code of professional conduct for nurses in 1983), nurses are known to have colluded in perpetrating what we would now consider to be betrayals of trust by health care professionals. Examples of such betrayals fill the pages of three particularly poignant and influential critiques of professional activity published between 1964 and 1984.[13] These texts detail example after example of institutionalised abuses of trust by health care professionals in the name of treatment and care of patients of all ages and capacities including, those with learning disabilities, children, the older person and the mentally ill.

Despite these shortcomings, which are by no means limited to the examples provided within the identified texts, there continues to be an enduring tradition that recognises (at least the rhetoric of) the importance of trust within relationships between health care professionals and patients. Indeed, part of the critique of the rise of institutional accountability in public service provision lies in a claim that the surveillance of audit occurs at the expense of trust relationships between professionals and clients (see, for example, O'Neill 2002; Smith 2001). It appears that the tradition of trust relationships as the cornerstone of health care provision has a long history of failing to protect *more-than-ordinarily* vulnerable persons. The assumption that patients ought to place their trust in doctors, nurses and others merely because they are qualified health care professionals is one that appears to lack any substantive foundation. Nevertheless, and despite a significant amount of evidence that health care professionals cannot always be trusted, there remains a willingness on the part of the general public to assume health care professionals can be trusted. It may be that what is needed, if health care professionals are to retain the idea that they should be trusted, is a commitment to becoming trustworthy practitioners and this necessitates an articulation of just what being trustworthy requires.

It should be evident from this brief overview that while the tradition of trust in health care can be the cornerstone of effective practice it does appear to be rather more open to abuse than many would wish it to be. In other words, the tradition of trust lacks sufficient substance to regulate practice where practitioners, with or without deliberate intent, assume the tradition to be self-regulating. As Kennedy notes, the harms that health care professionals do, do not necessarily arise from malevolence; harmful practices do sometimes result from the actions of well-intentioned individuals. In describing the failings of children's cardiac surgery services in Bristol, Kennedy states:

It is an account of people who cared greatly about human suffering, and were dedicated and well-motivated. Sadly, some lacked insight and their behaviour was flawed... Despite their manifest good intentions and long hours of dedicated work, there were failures on occasion in the care provided to very sick children. (Kennedy 2001, p.1)

Thus it might be thought that good will alone is an insufficient condition for trust but this would be to confuse good will with, for example, mere good intentions or dedication. While these (and other) things may well be important aspects, there is yet more to be said about quite what it is that a good will requires and we will come to this in due course. For now we must continue with our account of the place of trust in the practice of nursing.

Trust in nursing: personal or professional?

Despite her objections, O'Neill (2002) does nevertheless admit that good will may be central in some, but not all, cases of personal trust. Assuming that it is generally considered desirable that nurses have good will towards patients, and given that nursing practice inevitably requires patients to reveal, willingly or not, intimate personal details (details moreover that might not be revealed outside of a professional caring relationship) then it would seem that even O'Neill must accept good will on the part of the nurse as a desirable if not essential feature of the trust relationship between a nurse and a patient, if only because the nurse–patient relationship cannot be regarded without recognising that it contains at least some features of personal trust. As Baier notes it is because we require the assistance of others in 'looking after the things we most value...[that] we have no choice but to allow some others to be in a position to harm them' (Baier 1986, p.236). In other words we cannot escape the need to trust at least some others, and this must entail some aspects of personal trust. In contrast, Gilbert argues that personal trust has no place in nursing. He says 'The nature of trust structured within nurse-client relations is a form of impersonal trust for it has no commitment beyond the specific circumstances of the system...' (Gilbert 1998, p.1015). For Gilbert any talk of trust within nursing practice is merely one part of a system of performance (what he calls 'impression management') for monitoring nursing actions and for containing patient expectations. But in rejecting the possibility that nurses can enter into a relationship with patients that contains at least some elements of personal trust, Gilbert offers only an impoverished view of the potential for health care practitioners to enhance the capacity of *more-than-ordinarily* vulnerable persons to flourish. Given these two choices (which, by implication, reflect quite different perspectives of the nature of nursing) it would be surprising if most individuals did not wish nurse–patient relationships to approximate personal rather than impersonal trust.

Personal trust relationships: friendship

The paradigm case of personal trust is often taken to be friendship, and while friendships and nurse–patient relationships are different, both require elements of personal forms of trust if either is to be anything more than a mere impersonal business-like relationship. Friendship is generally considered to be a relationship that one freely chooses to enter and one in which trust develops over time to become a feature that defines the relationship as a friendship (although it should be apparent that there are different levels of friendship implying varying degrees of trust). Clearly, whatever the nurse–patient relationship is and however it develops, it does not share common origins with friendship for, generally speaking and at the point of first contact, patients do not freely choose to enter relationships with individual nurses. So it might seem from the outset that the project to locate such relationships in terms of personal trust has already run into serious difficulties. But while it is true that the nature of the relationship between patient and nurse is different from friendship it nevertheless remains the case that, except in rare instances, interactions between patients and nurses are, by their very nature, at least personal and sometimes intimate. Thus at this point it is with ideas of personal trust in mind that the inquiry proceeds.

De Raeve (2002) responds to a criticism advanced by, among others, MacIntyre that professionals (and by implication nurses) can only ever be inauthentic in their relationships with patients. This is to say that because professionals must necessarily modify their emotional responses they cannot lay claim to a genuine relationship with patients. Professionals can never respond only in the way that, for example, a friend can for this would be to compromise the professional–patient relationship. MacIntyre says:

> Sometimes…social workers are taught to become 'friends' with their clients in order to gain their confidence so as to manipulate them more effectively. Now it is of the essence of friendship as a virtue that one cannot become a friend from such a motive and with such an intention. (MacIntyre 1975, p.106)

By extension, De Raeve argues that nurses must respond to the charge that any trust relationship with a patient is founded on an untrustworthy and inauthentic premise of 'fake' interest in the well-being of that patient. De Raeve points out that to characterise the nurse–patient relationship as inauthentic on such grounds is to fail to recognise the relationship for what it is, and for the instrumental purpose(s) for which it exists. Or rather, it is to fail to recognise that a relationship between a nurse and a patient is essentially instrumental in origin but need not remain wholly instrumental. Indeed De Raeve, amongst others, would claim that a wholly instrumental relationship between a nurse and a patient would (generally speaking) be taken to be a poor example of professional nursing. The instrumental origin of the relationship does not, of itself, preclude authenticity in interactions between nurse and patient, and it does not mean that nurses are inherently untrustworthy (as MacIntyre implies). But what it does mean is that the trust relationship between a nurse and a patient is essentially different from that between friends (or from other sorts of everyday intimate relationships) and to judge them by the same criteria is inappropriate. In addition, in making his claim MacIntyre resorts to cynical characterisation of what it is that social workers might, sometimes, be taught. He also assumes too much in making two sub-claims: 1) that in claiming that sometimes social workers are taught to become friends to their clients, they are being taught to be friends with clients in the same way that they would become friends with individuals outside of a professional–client relationship (that is, in the sense of developing social friendships) and 2) that in becoming friends to clients there is an intention to manipulate those clients. Neither of these claims withstands close scrutiny. These claims cannot go unchallenged for to accept MacIntyre's characterisation of professional–client relationships is to accept that virtues play no part in the work of nurses (and other health and social care professionals); indeed, it is to accept that professionals misappropriate virtues for instrumental purposes and in so doing turn them into vices.

MacIntyre does not source his evidence for the claim but it is difficult to imagine that any curriculum (even one from the 1970s) would make any explicit statements of the sort that social workers should be taught to become friends with their clients. It is possible (even likely) that MacIntyre has misinterpreted the idea that in the 1970s social workers may have been encouraged to *befriend* their clients but this is an altogether different proposition. The idea of befriending clients (if, indeed, this idea is, or has been, encouraged by those who teach social workers) is quite different from the idea of becoming friends, and would be understood to be very different from friendship as such by social care professionals. The everyday meaning of befriending is, after all, to *act as a friend*, not to be a friend.

The claim that social workers are taught to become a friend *in order to manipulate the client* is highly speculative and rests on the interpretation of social work as state sponsored surveillance. It is true that social work, unlike nursing, is highly political but social workers are acutely aware of the possibility of being used as, or of being perceived as, agents of state control. This goes some way to explain the emphasis on values in social work education and the articulation of the aim of empowering disadvantaged individuals and groups in codes of practice for social workers (see, for example, Banks 2001).

These criticisms with which De Raeve takes issue might also be characterised as overly romanticising the idea of authentic relationships such as those between friends. It is true that one hopes one's friends to be one's friends for more than merely instrumental reasons but it would seem unreasonable for one's friends to have no instrumental gains from the friendship. In addition, it would also seem unreasonable to suppose that one's friends do not modify their emotional responses, for if one expects one's friends to repress their own interests in the interests of friendship it is, perhaps, to demand too much. Friends do modify their reactions to one another in order to maintain friendships. If it is to be said that friendships are genuine relationships despite modifications of emotional responses done for the good of the friendship then there would seem no reason not to apply the same logic to the nurse–patient relationship. One might therefore claim that the modifications of responses on the part of the nurse are equally genuine because those modifications aim at the good of the patient (however defined) and this would seem, at least prima facie, authentic. What would be inauthentic would be for a nurse to modify her or his responses for reasons that have nothing to do with promoting the well-being of a patient. This would also be to fail to engage with nursing as a practice as defined in Chapter 3.

Personal trust relationships: kinship

For some it is kinship rather than friendship that forms the paradigm case of personal trust. Fukuyama (1995) describes the cultural determinants of the boundaries of our trust relations when, for example, he contrasts the tendency of Chinese communities to consider trust to be limited to family with the European tradition of trusting non-family. He draws on Redding who states 'The key feature [of Hong Kong businesses] would appear to be that you trust your family absolutely, your friends and acquaintances to the degree that mutual dependence has been established... *With everybody else you make no assumptions about their goodwill*' (Redding 1990, p.66; emphasis added). While Fukuyama is using culturally determined differences in trust relations to illustrate differences in the development of businesses in different parts of the world his point readily translates to other social relationships. In addition both Fukuyama and Redding lend support to Baier's assertion of the relationship between good or ill will on one hand and trust on the other. In Baier's terms then, the assumption of Chinese communities is that few outside the family have good will toward one. In the European and North American tradition trust tends to be more readily located within friendships and this allows for an extended scope of trust that may go beyond the family, or may even supplant the family. The point here is that while we must all allow some others (trustworthy others we hope) to get close enough to harm us or the things we care about we nevertheless have discretion to choose which others we will so trust. Fukuyama's position would presumably be that we are in fact limited in our choice in trusting because of our cultural inheritance, but he would allow, I think, that our choices nevertheless rest on the idea that we will trust those whom we assume to have a good will towards us.

Trust relationships in nursing

Personal trust then comes as part of the choices that are available to us as we build trust relationships over time with those around us. However when becoming a patient our prior experiences of personal trust relationships do not necessarily provide us with the wherewithal to negotiate a world in which we have no control over, for example, which nurse will be looking after us. Which nurse, that is, who we must necessarily allow close enough to be in a position to harm us, whether we trust them or not. Nevertheless, if we are able to, we will continue to make instant judgements about those health care workers who present themselves as our carers. We may have a general dispositional distrust of institutions (which might well be misplaced mistrust) and might, therefore, not trust any health care professional with whom we come into contact; we may nevertheless be forced to rely on them. In sharp contrast we may trust all health care professionals as part of a faith in a background of trust in health care provision (which might be to misplace trust); indeed, there is some evidence of a blind trust tendency of patients (Thorne and Robinson 1988). If able, we may judge one nurse to be more worthy of our trust than another after only minimal contact reflecting our ability to make everyday judgements about the trustworthiness of others. As Baier remarks, 'before proceeding into the dark street or library stacks…[we] judge the few people…there to be nondangerous' (Baier 1986, p.237). In other words we quickly decide whether or not to trust the strangers with whom we come into contact. If we judge them to be disposed not to do us harm we will trust in this minimal formulation. If we judge them neither well nor ill disposed toward us we may still proceed although we are unlikely to trust them, rather we may rely on their willingness to conform to the normal social expectation of not unnecessarily interfering with us. If we judge them ill disposed toward us then we may decide that to proceed would be foolish and, if we have a choice in the matter, abandon our intent. If, however, we judge that they have an ill will toward us and we have no choice but to proceed then we can either hope that they will choose not to harm us, or rely on systems of surveillance to prevent them from harming us. This everyday experience of making rapid judgements about others' intentions towards us is something we take with us as patients. Under normal circumstances our initial impressions of the relative trustworthiness of others is likely to be both incomplete and in need of subsequent review as we learn more about those individual others. For as Potter notes 'When we want to determine whether or not to trust another with the care of some good we value, we need to know what the other's values, commitments, and loyalties are' (Potter 2002, p.7). In fact, if we have any choice in the matter at all, we express some form of background trust by allowing ourselves to become patients in the first place. Even if we have no choice and even if we believe we have good reason not to trust nurses we must either rely on the systems of accountability (that is, trust in institutions) that regulate nursing practice or merely hope that we will not be harmed by untrustworthy nurses.

Professional trust relationships

Thus, trust and trustworthiness are important in health care in general and in nursing in particular. This trust necessarily has elements of personal trust if nursing is conceived as anything other a mere impersonal business-type arrangement but, while some similarities exist, nursing cannot be categorised as an example of personal trust. Some instances of nursing practice may approximate personal trust because of the nature of the interventions required in particular situations. I am thinking here of the therapeutic relationships in some parts of nursing practice with persons suffering mental health issues, or those within learning disabilities nursing where anecdotal reports of friendships developed between nurses and service users are not uncommon. But these instances arise as a result of an initial professional–client relationship and such friendships as do develop, develop over and above this. Hence we might categorise trust in nursing as professional rather than personal trust. There is a tendency for trust to be categorised as trust in persons (personal trust) or trust in institutions[14] but trust in nursing seems not to fit either description.

The idea of professional trust offers a way of thinking about nurse–patient relationships that allows for elements of both trust in persons and trust in institutions. Nurses can be trusted (or not) both as individuals (with qualities we associate with personal trust) and as representatives of nursing as an institution (with, for example, a healthy dose of distrust under relevant circumstances). This recognises one tension for nurses in the face of sometimes competing demands: that is, tensions between the demands of the profession, the employer, the patient, the relatives of the patient and so on. One thing that acting as a professional requires is that each individual nurse must negotiate a way through tensions of this nature. These sorts of tensions seem to be an inevitable part of the work of nurses and are as relevant in matters of trust as any other aspect of a nurse's professional activity.

Competence and professional trust

It might be suggested that trust is not needed because reliable nurses and confidence in systems can assure safe care, but this would merely be a threshold of care. Of course, such a threshold of safe care is important in itself and if one had to choose between being cared for by a trustworthy yet incompetent nurse on the one hand or a competent but merely reliable nurse on the other one would tend to choose the latter for obvious reasons. Yet this categorisation is false for, as we shall see, a trustworthy nurse is one who is at a minimum both competent and reliable. So choices might be more accurately described in a different way. One choice might be between the incompetent and the competent nurse and one would normally choose the competent nurse in order to ensure a threshold level of care; this together with reliable systems to ensure practising nurses are competent serves to inspire confidence in nursing as an institution. Thus the minimum requirement for reliance is met. A second choice, if there is one, might be between a merely competent nurse and a trustworthy nurse. This distinction is one that hinges on the character of the nurse and on her or his propensity to engage with nursing as a practice (as defined in Chapter 3). It is unlikely that when one becomes a patient one will know very much about the character of the nurse(s) providing care so at this point one may either rely on one's confidence in the system of health care or make a rapid initial judgement about the trustworthiness of the nurse.

Thus confidence in the system to provide reliable and competent nurses offers a threshold of safe care and this is important for those who find themselves in receipt of nursing practice. It provides the basis from which trust might emerge (although this need not be a necessary condition). Nevertheless, an account of nurse–patient relationships based on mere reliance, rather than on trust, remains unsatisfactory because trust and trustworthiness contribute to human flourishing in more convincing ways than do mere reliance and confidence, and it should be said, in more satisfying ways than do mere belief or hope. The idea of care provided without some conception of trust and therefore in the absence of good will is not one that appeals even in acute emergency life saving circumstances. And if one legitimate aim of nursing is, as I have claimed, the flourishing of *more-than-ordinarily* vulnerable persons then the dispositions that nurses should have are those dispositions that encourage human flourishing. And trustworthiness is one such disposition. That a nurse should be trustworthy is of particular importance for those *more-than-ordinarily* vulnerable persons who, for whatever reason, are not in a position to assess the trustworthiness of others.

Independent practical reasoning and trust

If the placing of trust hinges on the cognitive capacities of the one trusting as assumed in a number of accounts of trust in nursing (for example, Gilbert 1998; Johns 1996; Meize-Grochowski 1984) then those with compromised or diminished cognitive capabilities cannot be said to trust. This idea is reflected in MacIntyre's requirement for independent practical reasoning if one is to trust but, as stated earlier, this is a contingent rather than absolute requirement. Thus while it may, on occasion, be true it cannot be generalised beyond some very limited cases. Some individuals may be unable to hold a belief as such (for example, an unconscious person cannot hold beliefs in the sense we usually understand people to hold, or act upon, beliefs) and therefore it is not possible for them to trust, although others may trust on their behalf. But those who lack a capacity (temporarily or permanently) to make an assessment of another's good will towards them may still be in a position to trust, even if this cannot be articulated in any formal sense. Contra Gilbert (1998) who claims that because trust involves choice what we observe in the absence of choice is hope rather than trust, Baier makes a case for infant trust representing fundamental trust as a state of nature. She says, convincingly, that 'surviving infants will usually have shown some trust, enough to accept offered nourishment' (Baier 1986, p.241). This inclination of an infant to trust suggests that trust, rather than distrust (certainly rather than mere hope) is the default position. It suggests a tendency to anticipate good will towards one, which later becomes fixed on particular others. So for the trusting infant, a trustworthy parent (or other carer) is the ideal if the child is to flourish. Similarly, for the trusting patient, a trustworthy nurse is a moral imperative especially where the recipient of nursing practice has a diminished or compromised capacity to make an assessment of the trustworthiness of others. Such patients are otherwise exposed to the possibility that those in whose care they are placed do not have a good will, indeed, may even have ill will, toward them. Being an untrustworthy nurse then is to fail to care for important human goods, the sorts of goods that, if we are able to, we value as goods essential for human flourishing. Thus abuse of trust of *more-than-ordinarily* vulnerable persons, especially those with a limited capacity to choose to trust, is fundamentally at odds with any conception of nursing that encompasses the good of the patient as an aim or as a good of practice. If this is true then it is to the trustworthiness of individual health care professionals rather than to the capacity of patients to exercise discretion in trusting that we must turn.

Trustworthiness

Rising to the challenge set by Baier who notes that 'One might have… expected those with a moral theory of the virtues to have looked at trustworthiness' (Baier 1986, p.232), Nancy Potter offers an account of trustworthiness as a virtue. Following Aristotle, Potter locates trustworthiness as a mean situated between insufficient care on one hand and an inappropriate and excessive way of caring for those things that others value on the other. She writes:

> *A trustworthy person…is one who can be counted on, as a matter of the sort of person he or she is, to take care of those things that others entrust to one and…whose ways of caring are neither excessive nor deficient…* An excess…might be the lack of discretion as to the limits to what one can reasonably care for or the lack of discretion as to appropriate objects of care… A deficiency…might be when one cannot be entrusted to properly care for what others value. (Potter 2002, pp.16–17; original emphasis)

Potter's account is a welcome contribution to a literature that is otherwise sparse in analyses of trustworthiness in general and the trustworthiness of health care professionals in particular. To my knowledge, Potter is the first to claim trustworthiness as a virtue. She notes that while it does not appear on Aristotle's list, the idea of trustworthiness as a character virtue is consistent with an Aristotelian account of the virtues. She notes further and with some accuracy, that there is a general agreement (albeit with caveats) on the moral value of trustworthiness. If trustworthiness is a virtue then it has been too long neglected and Potter has done us a service in beginning the discussion. However, one of the difficulties in conceiving of trustworthiness as a virtue (and possibly a reason that it has not been claimed as a virtue previously) is that it differs from the standard requirements of a virtue insofar as it is particularly susceptible to situation. It is not merely that different interpretations of trustworthiness are likely, for this is true of other, accepted, virtues such as courage. Rather it is that the degree to which someone is considered to be trustworthy will depend upon the perspectives of those placing (or misplacing) trust. So whereas both friend and foe can agree on the courageousness of a soldier in battle, in situations of trust involving more that one other person conflict is always a possibility and the same action that upholds the trust of one party may be betrayal for another. This is because in being trustworthy we choose both an allegiance and a moral stance in relation to others.

Potter claims that being untrustworthy is sometimes the trustworthy thing to do. For example, in betraying an undertaking not to inform the authorities when an acquaintance confesses to abusing his child one has made a moral choice between breaking the trust of an acquaintance rather than that of his child. Whatever one does in a situation of this kind there will be at least one third party who will perceive one's act (or omission) as an act of betrayal, a betrayal of trust and, as such, one becomes, even if only for a single instance, untrustworthy *from that person's point of view*. This extreme illustration serves to highlight a tension in the notion of trustworthiness although it might be said that in the situation as described the trust placed by the acquaintance is illegitimate and hence cannot be a trust betrayed. Indeed, it might be said that were such a confidence given to a dispositionally trustworthy person, that person is to be trusted to act in a way that is trustworthy from the child's perspective because they understand the immorality of child abuse. Maybe so, but the example is meant only to illustrate a point that might be captured better by a less extreme example. Potter notes that what she calls 'mid level' workers (a category in which she includes nurses) often find themselves trusted from a number of different perspectives. So in matters of being worthy of trust a nurse might find themselves judged by, amongst others, a doctor, a nurse administrator, a nursing professional body, as well as by a patient or a patient's wife, father, mother, child and so on, each of whom may have a different expectation of what it means to be a trustworthy nurse. The patient may trust the nurse to tell him the truth about his condition, the patient's wife may trust the nurse to conceal the diagnosis from her husband, a doctor may trust the nurse to carry out his instructions, the nurse administrator may trust the nurse to follow protocol, and the professional body may trust the nurse to comply with their professional nursing code. It may be that each of these trust expectations might be reasonable in particular circumstances, yet if the patient has not been informed that he has cancer, if his wife has asked the doctor not to let the patient discover the diagnosis, if the doctor 'orders' the nurse not to tell the patient, if the hospital protocol is that nurses should follow medical instructions and if the nursing codes indicates that nurses should be honest in their dealings with patients then it should be clear that, whatever the nurse does, one or more of those involved will judge the nurse to have been untrustworthy. And this will be the case regardless of any general disposition the nurse may have in regard towards being trustworthy. Without a simplistic or deontological view of who one should be trustworthy towards and given the sorts of tensions in professional life as outlined above, the idea of a trustworthy nurse is far from straightforward. Apart from the difficulty in working out to whom one should be trustworthy in any given situation, the idea that a nurse should have or should cultivate a trustworthy character seems to rely on a conception of an ideal practice environment in which failures of trust reside in individual nurses. The reality of practice is such that to claim failures of trust are solely failures of character is to neglect the effects of both institutional activities and complex professional relationships.

Potter's account of trustworthiness as a virtue

Potter offers an account of trustworthiness as a virtue outlined within the framework of ten requirements for 'full trustworthiness'. Full trustworthiness here is contrasted with the trustworthiness of particular situations. Hence one can be trustworthy in particular instances or towards particular persons without necessarily being dispositionally trustworthy. This distinction is important for Potter who believes it necessary to distinguish these as two different types of trustworthiness. For Potter this means that being trustworthy in relation to specific tasks or people is not, of itself, a virtue. On this account trustworthiness is only a virtue when being trustworthy in specific situations reflects a genuine disposition of general trustworthiness.

Potter's ten requirements for full trustworthiness

1. That we give signs and assurances of our trustworthiness.

2. That we take our epistemic responsibility seriously.

3. That we develop sensitivity to the particularities of others.

4. That we respond properly to broken trust.

5. That we deal with hurt in relationships – both the hurt we inflict on others and the hurt we experience from others – in ways that sustain connection.

6. That our institutions and governing bodies be virtuous.

7. That we recognize the importance of being trustworthy to the disenfranchised and oppressed.

8. That we are committed to mutuality in intimate as well as in civic relationships.

9. That we work to sustain connection in intimate relationships while neither privatizing nor endangering mutual flourishing.

10. That we need also to have other virtues.

(Potter 2002, pp.26–31)

As Potter notes, the list of requirements presupposes 'a genuine regard for the good of others' (2002, p.31). Thus she seems to indicate that the virtue of trustworthiness requires a positive injunction for good will towards others, rather than merely a lack of ill will. These conditions are demanding and make full trustworthiness difficult to achieve but this is something it shares with other character dispositions. To assess the reasonableness (or otherwise) of Potter's requirements each of these conditions will be outlined in turn.

1. THAT WE GIVE SIGNS AND ASSURANCES OF OUR TRUSTWORTHINESS

As suggested above, it is likely that in attempting to be trustworthy health care professionals may find themselves pulled in different directions. That a nurse must sometimes choose between different trust expectations and therefore betray someone's trust seems inevitable. But in choosing whose trust to betray the nurse is demonstrating an allegiance. This might tell us something about the character of that nurse but a display of loyalty in one situation cannot be assumed to be symptomatic of a generalised disposition of trustworthiness towards a particular individual or group. Nevertheless, it is to be assumed that inferences will be made by those who witness a betrayal of trust about the likelihood of future trustworthy or untrustworthy behaviour by that particular nurse. This is what I take Potter to mean in claiming this first of her requirements of trustworthiness: giving *signs and assurances of our trustworthiness* (p.27; original emphasis). It is not that we must ask people to trust us, for as Baier (1986) reminds us such an injunction means little: others will either already believe us to be trustworthy, in which case the statement is redundant, or believe us to be untrustworthy, in which case the words alone will do little to convince them otherwise. In asking us to make known our trustworthiness Potter requires a demonstration of this trustworthiness. The signs and assurances she seeks are those that enable others to see that we have a good will towards them, that when we are entrusted with the things they value we will care for them in a way that respects and recognises their value to this particular individual at this particular point in time. It is a demonstration that we will not exploit their weaknesses or vulnerabilities. It is in deeds rather than in rhetoric that we prove ourselves to be trustworthy.

2. THAT WE TAKE OUR EPISTEMIC RESPONSIBILITY SERIOUSLY

Potter takes this to be a requirement for reflection and self-knowledge. To be trustworthy one needs to know what effect one has on others, how one's own moral values and beliefs can be perceived by others and the relationship this has to one's trustworthiness from the perspective of those others. It is to engage with the question: How do I know I am trustworthy? According to Potter, assumptions about one's own trustworthiness can be unreliable, particularly in relation to people with different social or cultural norms. It may come as a surprise for a western male health care worker to find himself apparently not trusted by, for example, a female Muslim patient. Such a surprise would only occur if the male health care worker had not taken his epistemic responsibilities seriously. Self-knowledge in identifying his own assumed trustworthiness as predicated on a set of social norms that not everyone shares will make it possible for him to recognise a need to be proactive in demonstrating his trustworthiness beyond the confines of his own social and cultural norms.

While Potter makes an important point here it is also necessary for a health care worker to take seriously the epistemic requirements of her or his particular role. That is, in order to be trustworthy the health care professional must know those things that are necessary for, at the very least, the competent practice of the particular skill(s) required of the role. It may be that Potter assumes this requirement for she notes elsewhere that as patients we need to exercise epistemic trust as well as general trust if we are to trust wisely when it comes to trusting health care professionals. In other words, if patients are to trust, they need to trust health care professionals to have the knowledge and skills necessary to provide safe, appropriate and competent health care. This requires that to be trustworthy health care professionals must ensure they retain the appropriate knowledge and skills and must not, for example, allow their knowledge to become out of date or allow their skills to deteriorate; these things require self-knowledge and self-awareness. Failure in either respect is to betray the trust invested in the individual acting in the role of health care professional. It requires a certain humility and open-mindedness which I take to be part of a good will towards others (that is, to be part of what it means to be trustworthy), for to allow one's knowledge to be insufficient or out of date, and to allow one's skills to become less than competent is to show a lack of good will towards patients, or in Potter's terms, a lack of regard for the good of others.

3. THAT WE DEVELOP SENSITIVITY TO THE PARTICULARITIES OF OTHERS

In her third requirement Potter suggests an essential component of full trustworthiness is the need to understand, from the perspective of the trusting person, the meaning and value of what it is they are entrusting. This requires both the epistemic effort of identifying the biases in one's assumed trustworthiness and of recognising that the trusting person is more than merely a member of a specific social or cultural group. It requires an attempt to grasp the significance *for that particular individual* of allowing others to be in a position to harm whatever it is they have entrusted. Thus, for nurses, a lack of sensitivity to the particularity of others would be demonstrated by treating patients merely as routine cases of a particular ailment, and referring to them (as was common practice in the 1960s) as, for example, the appendicectomy in bed five. Talking and thinking about persons in this way has been discredited (although vestiges of the practice remain in some areas) because it fails to recognise that, despite common features of conditions, individuals react both physically and emotionally in different ways to illness. The significance of a leg amputation is likely to be different for a footballer than for a bank clerk (although neither will find it trivial) and this is because of their particular circumstances. Developing a sensitivity to the particularities of others assists in aiming for the mean in being trustworthy. Without it there is a risk of failing to be trustworthy by acting in ways that neglect the importance to the one doing the trusting of that which they have entrusted (and we may do this either by not meeting or by exceeding in inappropriate ways the requirements of full trustworthiness).

4. THAT WE RESPOND PROPERLY TO BROKEN TRUST

Potter describes a situation in which a health care worker, having given assurances to the contrary, lies to a client in order to save her life. While recognising that moral theory and bioethics can provide persuasive reasons justifying a lie in the sorts of circumstances she describes, there remains a tendency, says Potter, for the matter to be left there. It is as if, she says, once an otherwise objectionable action is justified there is nothing more to be said. Potter notes, with some accuracy, that this is often not the end of the matter for the individual health care worker who delivered the lie (or other deception) or for the individual client whose trust has been betrayed. It is to this general neglect of character in bioethics that Potter takes exception. In her example the health care worker has betrayed the trust of the patient, and has, at least in a single instance, proved untrustworthy having claimed to be trustworthy. Her objection is that even when the breaking of a trust is the 'right thing' to do it nevertheless leaves those health care workers who take trustworthiness to be important in their relationships with patients in an invidious position. For Potter then, a further requirement for someone who is fully trustworthy (someone, that is, who has the virtue of trustworthiness) is that following a breach of trust not only will they know and feel that harm has occurred but that they will attempt to make reparation. The form of this reparation will depend on a number of factors but will be at a minimum an apology and an explanation with the aim of recovering trust. However, as noted earlier, trust is fragile and the recovery of a trust lost is not an easy matter, and while attempts to restore trust might offer something tangible to the one who broke the trust (for example, the attempt to make reparation, whether successful or not, might merely serve to ease the conscience of the betrayer of trust), it may do little for the one who has experienced betrayal.

5. THAT WE DEAL WITH HURT IN RELATIONSHIPS – BOTH THE HURT WE INFLICT ON OTHERS AND THE HURT WE EXPERIENCE FROM OTHERS – IN WAYS THAT SUSTAIN CONNECTION

In this requirement Potter begins to outline her sociological assumptions, for she recognises that hurt in relationships occurs beyond the realms of trust and trustworthiness. In terms of the hurt we cause, she places emphasis on two points. The first is that in betraying trust, whether intentional or not, we inflict hurt, and trustworthiness requires us to both notice the hurt caused and attempt to make amends. The second is the more general point that in noticing the ways in which we cause hurt (whether or not this is in terms of betraying trust) being trustworthy requires us to set about cultivating our habits so as to reduce the hurt we inflict. In other words, this is a general injunction to become a better person by improving our character. Improving our character also allows us to develop appropriate ways to respond to the hurt that others cause us so that we do not become isolated.

Dealing with hurt then means that when we attempt to make reparation to those we have hurt, we accept responsibility for inflicting that hurt and acknowledge that we may need to work hard to restore trust (and sometimes expect to suffer hurt ourselves in the process). Nevertheless, while it might be appropriate in general to aim for sustaining connection when dealing with hurt in relationships, Potter seems not to acknowledge that it is likely that there will be occasions when sustaining connections in both professional and personal relationships will impede rather than enable flourishing. Recognising when attempts to sustain connections no longer contribute to human flourishing is surely a necessary co-requirement of dealing with hurt in relationships, although professional accountability may well preclude abandoning connection in many professional relationships.

6. THAT OUR INSTITUTIONS AND GOVERNING BODIES BE VIRTUOUS

The betrayal of trust in Potter's case study (see requirement 4 above) takes place during a crisis intervention and once the services of the crisis centre are no longer required, further contact with the client is not possible. This means that in this instance the health care worker who betrayed the trust placed in her is unable to take any steps to repair the broken trust. This leads Potter to conclude that full trustworthiness requires suitable institutional arrangements and these will be found most often in the virtuous institution. A point which is made forcefully by MacIntyre (1985) who notes the modern tension between practices and institutions, and that, while the virtues may flourish within practices, because practices depend for their survival on institutions, it is the institutions that will determine the extent to which the virtues can flourish within practices. A virtuous institution is one in which individuals are encouraged to cultivate the virtues and to act in virtuous ways. To put this another way, if it is believed that practitioners should act virtuously then institutional arrangements must reduce tensions of the sort described earlier and in requirement 7 (below).

7. THAT WE RECOGNIZE THE IMPORTANCE OF BEING TRUSTWORTHY TO THE DISENFRANCHISED AND OPPRESSED

Essential to this seventh requirement of Potter's is the notion that in deciding to whom one should be trustworthy it is important to recognise that many patients and clients have already suffered the effects of trust betrayals (in some cases many times over). Potter takes a largely feminist political stance in arguing that social and institutional structures (in North America) tend to favour white middle-class males and that this predominant bias does little to engender the trust of those who do not fit the existing hegemony. Neither, to return to requirement 2 above, does it encourage those who are part of the dominant class to question their assumptions about their own trustworthiness. Hence, for Potter, anyone who is not part of the dominant group will already have reason to be cautious about the claims to trustworthiness of authority figures. She says:

The nature of trustworthiness is nonexploitative and nondominating. As such, exhibiting this virtue demands that, when we face conflicts with regard to whom to sustain or break trusting relations, we take as a primary consideration those who are already vulnerable in relation to dominant structures, in general, and to us, in particular. (Potter 2002, p.29)

For nurses, then, this requires the assumption that it should be the patient's trust one should maintain; it requires that we presume a patient's trust should be broken when, and only when, there are compelling reasons to do so. Betraying the trust of a patient without a compelling reason is to exploit their position of vulnerability. The patient is, so to speak, an easy option when conflicts of trust cannot be avoided for, generally speaking, within the health care system it is the patient who is least likely to know what is going on. Those working within the institutions and practices of health care have a knowledge and understanding of the health care system, the advantages and disadvantages of particular forms of treatment and care, and a way of evaluating service delivery usually denied to those who are the recipients of that care. Hence patients are already vulnerable in respect of health care professionals and institutions, and to add to that vulnerability by betrayal(s) of trust is to compound disadvantage. For those who are already further disadvantaged by the fact of compromised or diminished rational capacities, betrayals of trust appear to be even more culpable.

8. THAT WE ARE COMMITTED TO MUTUALITY IN INTIMATE AS WELL AS IN CIVIC RELATIONSHIPS

Potter's account starts to become sketchy at this point but she seems to use the term mutuality to mean something like a willingness to cooperate with others on the basis of trusting relationships. Hence mutual relationships both rely on and sustain trust whereas 'Nonmutual relationships are untrustworthy ones and so impede flourishing' (Potter 2002, p.30). Because Potter's idea of 'nonmutuality' is insufficiently developed it is difficult to be sure what makes a relationship nonmutual beyond a general idea of non-cooperation. However, she does claim that mutuality in relationships allows us to challenge covert and overt power relationships, which in turn assists the project of reducing exploitation and abuse of vulnerable persons. Further, she claims that nonmutuality in relationships provides an opportunity for distrust to thrive, thereby reducing the potential for human flourishing.

9. THAT WE WORK TO SUSTAIN CONNECTION IN INTIMATE RELATIONSHIPS WHILE NEITHER PRIVATIZING NOR ENDANGERING MUTUAL FLOURISHING

Following on from requirement 8 above, Potter notes that intimate relationships engender a depth of trust (and trustworthiness) beyond that required for normal everyday trust relationships. She argues that by experiencing the depth of intimate trusting relationships we can add to the sum of human flourishing as it enables us to become generally more trusting and trustworthy (and therefore enables a commitment to mutuality). She suggests this is important for professional trust relationships because our experience of 'deep' trust spills over into and informs both our general and professional trust dispositions. The experience of deep trust in intimate relationships gives us insights into the nature of trust and trustworthiness by placing us in positions of vulnerability, it helps us to reflect on our own as well as on others' willingness to trust, and it enables us to recognise how painful betrayals of trust can be. If we know what it is to be vulnerable in this way then we can better appreciate the vulnerability of those who must trust in health care professionals. From this we are more likely to recognise the need to be trustworthy towards those in the most vulnerable positions, that is, our patients and clients.

However, while sustaining connection may be appropriate for 'healthy' intimate relationships, Potter seems to fail to recognise the reality that some people experience 'unhealthy' intimate relationships. Working to maintain such relationships seems likely to impede rather than enable flourishing. It must surely be more appropriate in terms of human flourishing to abandon rather than sustain 'unhealthy' intimate relationships.

10. THAT WE NEED ALSO TO HAVE OTHER VIRTUES

Potter argues here for an Aristotelian unity of the virtues. She says 'trustworthiness is part of a family of virtues that require the development of other-regarding or altruistic dispositions and that each of the virtues is necessary for the full expression of the rest' (p.31). It is this point that leads her to conclude that to be trustworthy one must have a concern for the well-being of other people that is not only authentic but is also expressed in one's actions and reactions (both physical and emotional) to the situations in which people find themselves. Although she does not provide a full list of the other virtues in this family of other-regarding virtues, it is clear that she takes her cue from Blum's (1980) discussion of the altruistic emotions, and includes 'thoughtfulness, beneficence, justice and compassion' (p.32) as likely candidates.

Discussion of Potter's account

Potter offers us a useful framework for thinking about the nature of trustworthiness, from which it may be possible to determine the extent to which someone is fully trustworthy. This assumes, of course, both that trustworthiness is a virtue and that Potter's ten requirements provide a comprehensive account.

Potter's ten requirements

Potter's intention in outlining the ten requirements seems to be both to offer a guide to the demands of 'full' trustworthiness and to judge the trustworthiness of a given individual. I have already offered some critical comments while outlining each of her requirements but the question of how far these ten requirements actually provide a comprehensive account remains. In one sense this project is doomed to fail as there is always likely to be occasion when being fully trustworthy requires us to act in ways that cannot be predicted. Indeed, if trustworthiness is a virtue then it would be unusual to expect that a set of comprehensive criteria for establishing its expression could be compiled. The general Aristotelian assumption would be that the expression of a virtue is measured against the good and against what a person with the virtues would do in those particular circumstances rather than by a set of artificially constructed criteria. But this may be to misinterpret Potter's intent. A more sympathetic reading might suggest that listing the ten requirements is an attempt to identify how demanding being trustworthy is and to offer us nothing more than a guide to how we might go about fulfilling an aspiration to be trustworthy. In this sense Potter's ten requirements offer us much of value to think about if we wish to cultivate a disposition of trustworthiness, if we wish, that is, to cultivate the virtue of trustworthiness.

Potter's critique of modern moral theory

Potter characterises modern ethical theory as unsympathetic to matters of character and certainly there is anecdotal evidence to support this assertion at least within medical and bioethics literature. There is no doubt that the principle-based approach of Beauchamp and Childress (2008) has come to dominate both the practice and the literature of medical and bioethics and some commentators argue that this does indeed give prominence to abstract reasoning. This seems to have led to a dominance of what might be termed a justification-oriented ethics where the emphasis of justification on the basis of abstract principles marginalises other more individual patient-oriented approaches. Indeed, this aspect of Potter's attack on modern moral theory can be read as part of a larger feminist critique of principlism. In this respect actions based on what Potter terms mainstream modern moral theory (and she really means, I think, medicine's interpretation of principlism as abstract rather than person-situated) do seem to leave the effects of such actions on individuals to one side when decisions are being made.

In reframing questions of justification from the perspective of what she understands as mainstream modern ethical theory to that of character virtues Potter addresses one of the very real tensions in health care practice: the tension practitioners experience when faced with real life dilemmas for which putative theoretical 'right actions' may well satisfy the requirements of rational argument but yet leave the practitioner finding the solution both unconvincing and unsatisfactory. In her example of telling a justified lie[15] to save a life, she reminds us that we remain in danger of harming ourselves as moral agents (we become untrustworthy, even if only on the one occasion) as well as those to whom we have lied (potentially affecting their future willingness-to-trust). Her claim is that modern moral theory as understood by doctors and administrators takes a short-term and narrow-minded view of the consequences of a justified lie, neglecting other morally significant effects of lying on both the perpetrator and the recipient of the lie. For Potter the most pernicious other morally significant effect is the effect on trusting relationships, both in specific cases and in general. If health care professionals accept betrayals of patients' trust as inevitable then claims to ethical practice ring somewhat hollow. Treating betrayals of trust as routine (on grounds provided by a narrow view of modern ethical theory) without recognising the potential this has to undermine not only professional trust relationships but also the general level background trust is to take a parochial view of health care practice. This is one of the central points in Janet Jackson's book-long argument 'explain[ing] why we need to adopt a very strict teaching repudiating the telling of lies…in medical and nursing practice' (Jackson 2001, p.ix). Thus Potter places the virtues and particularly the virtue of trustworthiness at the heart of matters in health care ethics. In so doing, trustworthiness becomes the focus for her analysis of the relationships between health care professionals and those for whom they provide care. What she finds is that while some harms are avoided by the application of mainstream modern moral theory (narrowly conceived), other potential harms are neglected. And it is these other harms that form part of the concerns of nurses who have found the practice of deception uncomfortable, even when putative moral justification has been provided. My own experience of facilitating discussions of ethical issues with qualified nurses reinforces this as they express similar concerns when they find themselves capitulating to or colluding with deceptions they find to be distressing. These concerns lend weight to Potter's claims about the failure of the modern application of moral theory; a failure to account for the moral sensibilities of the actors involved. While the attempt to remove emotion from ethics by concentrating on abstract reasoning can provide justification for some otherwise morally objectionable practices, it rarely (if ever) provides sufficiently consistent (or acceptable) logical conclusions at the extremes without some tortuous form of convoluted argumentation or the application of some additional principle. Attempts to pick out inconsistencies and counter argument are, after all, what fill the pages of bioethics texts and journals.

Nursing takes place within institutional contexts grounded in artificial and bureaucratic constructions; an environment in which it is possible, should one so choose, to divorce one's professional life from one's personal life. In such an environment it becomes easy to imagine that decisions made in the professional arena are unrelated to the social world. This separation between the professional and the personal provides the possibility for the corruption of character of those who wish to engage with ethical practice, especially in the face of established and dominant justificatory, but incomplete, rationales for right actions. This is one of the reasons that Potter argues for the need for virtuous institutions, that is, institutions with arrangements that enable practitioners to express rather than suppress the virtues.

As indicated earlier, those who practice as nurses often find themselves in situations that are different from normal social conventions; or rather, practising nurses find themselves working in environments where the normal patterns of acceptable moral behaviour may be substantively different from those of everyday life and for which it appears everyday life provides insufficient preparation. In everyday social situations people are not usually confronted by others whose suffering is such that were it seen in a horse, dog or cat would lead to those animals being 'put down'. And what seems to be acceptable moral behaviour in respect of non-human animals cannot be merely transferred into the environment in which health care takes place. Thus, generally speaking, when individuals begin to practise nursing they are unprepared to deal with the sorts of dilemmas with which they will become confronted. A general disposition to be just, honest, courageous or trustworthy might provide a secure foundation *in most cases* for moral actions in the everyday world and such everyday virtues *might serve as a basis* for moral behaviour in the professional practice of nursing, but they will not necessarily be sufficient to enable a nurse to act as a virtuous agent. It is often claimed that nursing is a moral endeavour as almost every action a nurse can take there is an alternative action omitted (Sellman 1996; Tschudin 1992), in part because there is always more for a nurse to do than can be done in the time available. So for a nurse to prioritise her or his time requires a consideration of her or himself as a finite resource the allocation of which equates with the identification of a greater value to one action, or to one patient, rather than another. So while a nurse may wish to practise in a just way, this may not be possible if the demands on the nurse are greater than her or his capacity to respond to those demands. Clearly, there is a sense in which virtue for nursing practice is different from general virtue. In the normal everyday world to act in accord with general virtue allows for the fact that one already has made some value judgements about one's sphere of responsibility. Normally, it is to one's family and friends, and perhaps to one's colleagues that one assumes specific obligations of general virtue together with a general lack of vice to others. Whereas a nurse who wishes to practice in accordance with the everyday virtues of truthfulness, courage and justice will find her or himself faced with dilemmas posed by those very virtues precisely because she or he is not normally able to select the boundaries of either the patients in her or his care or the demands those patients will make.

The professional virtue of trustworthiness

I suggested earlier that it may be wise to reserve judgement on the question of whether or not trustworthiness is a virtue. While the idea of the virtues has a tradition that predates Aristotle there remains contention about the exact nature of virtue. It is not my intention to enter this particular debate; it is mentioned merely in passing to acknowledge the definitional difficulties. How then are we to assess the claims of one or other writer that such and such is a virtue? One feature consistent with my brief sketch of virtue in Chapter 1 (and with an Aristotelian account of the virtues) is that a virtue is a more or less permanent disposition from which an agent is guided to act in ways that encourage rather than discourage human flourishing.[16] In this respect, especially with Potter's emphasis on its relationship with human flourishing, trustworthiness looks like a candidate for being classed as a virtue. However, as I noted at the beginning of this section, there are tensions involved in being trustworthy that may preclude it from being a virtue. The capacity to be trustworthy is not in question (although, as Potter notes, one may not be the best judge of one's own trustworthiness) rather it is that it seems to be possible for an act to be both trustworthy and untrustworthy at the same time. This is to be contrasted with virtues such as honesty and courage where the assessment of a person's honesty or courage does not change depending upon their relationship with others. It is not possible to be both truthful and untruthful at the same time, even if some others would rather not hear the truth. A judgement about one's honesty relies on an assessment of correspondence between reality and what one says (assuming that is one is convinced by correspondence theories of truth), and this is so regardless of who is making that judgement. Furthermore, and leaving aside the capacity to fool oneself, self-assessment of one's honesty is relatively straightforward. In contrast, the assessment of one's trustworthiness is complicated by the necessity to decide to whom one should be trustworthy. However, just as Williams (2002) claims that there are *virtues* (rather than a single virtue) of truthfulness, and MacIntyre (1999) talks of the *virtues* of independent practical reason, it may be that we should think of the *virtues* of trustworthiness.

It is not yet clear that trustworthiness can take its place alongside established virtues, particularly in the light of the foregoing discussion. However, no conception of virtue is without difficulty, and for some (including Potter) a virtue approach offers the best alternative to the unresolved (perhaps even irresolvable) problems that beset modern moral theory. It might be more productive to consider trustworthiness against other virtues. The virtue of justice may share some of these relational difficulties. There are a number of conceptions of justice and the difficulties this presents are compounded by the use of the term justice in ethical thought; some use justice to describe an ethical principle (indeed, it is a core principle in the major versions of principle-based ethics); others use it to mean a virtue; others conflate the two suggesting that it can serve as both principle and virtue.

For Aristotle, justice requires that we do not differentiate our responses to others on irrelevant grounds; a sentiment that meets with almost universal approval. MacIntyre (1985) reinforces the point by noting that it would be unjust for a professor to award grades on the basis of, for example, some arbitrary whim or some particular distinction over which the student has no control (such as the colour of his eyes). Justice demands that we assess student essays on the basis of merit. A student may, of course, *perceive* that his work has been judged unjustly, and in this respect justice seems to share a problem familiar to trustworthiness. That is, the same act *can* be judged to be just by one person and unjust by another, in the same way that a single act can be judged trustworthy and untrustworthy from the perspective of different persons. Yet there is a significant difference, for if the professor awards marks on the basis of merit then she will not be struggling with the sort of dilemma the nurse in our earlier example is experiencing in deciding to whom she should be trustworthy. In marking students' assignments, the professor can be either just or unjust, but not both at the same time (regardless of the conception of justice held), whereas our nurse knows that whatever action she or he chooses, a betrayal of trust will occur.

It is not clear that these problems are sufficient to claim trustworthiness cannot be a virtue. Indeed, if Aristotle is correct in noting that aiming to do the right thing to the right person in the right way at the right time and for the right reason is what helps us towards the expression of virtue then we may yet find that we are fully trustworthy (that is, we express the virtue of trustworthiness) if and only if we have identified the right person to whom we should be trustworthy. Thus it might be that trustworthiness is indeed a virtue in its own right. While there is yet more to be said about this matter my tentative conclusion is that trustworthiness might well be a virtue especially given that trustworthiness has such a prominent place in promoting human flourishing. In any case, there is no doubt that we can accept trustworthiness as a desirable professional virtue for it should be clear from the foregoing discussion that if nurses are serious about caring for *more-than-ordinarily* vulnerable persons as part of a commitment to human flourishing then being trustworthy (from the perspective of patients) is a necessary condition of practice.

5 Open-mindedness

Thus far I have argued that in addition to the virtues of honesty, justice and courage the professional virtue of trustworthiness is essential for nursing conceived as a practice in the technical sense that MacIntyre uses that term. Where full virtue is not possible (and I have provided some reasons why full virtue might not be possible) then these dispositions must be expressed in a minimal formulation as professional virtues. The importance of trust and trustworthiness cannot be over-emphasised, yet there are components of the professional virtue of trustworthiness about which more must yet be said. One such feature identified by Potter (2002) and discussed briefly in Chapter 4 is the need to understand the epistemic requirements of being trustworthy as a nurse. In this chapter one aspect of these epistemic responsibilities, the need to be dispositionally open-minded, is discussed. Open-mindedness is regarded as a necessary professional virtue for the practice of nursing. Aiming towards being dispositionally open-minded contributes to the maintenance of epistemic responsibilities by helping nurses to avoid becoming either closed-minded or credulous. These two failures of open-mindedness have the potential not only to corrupt the practice of nursing but also to make more difficult the task of nursing; that is to say that a failure of open-mindedness on the part of a nurse is likely to hinder rather than enable the flourishing of *more-than-ordinarily* vulnerable persons.

Open-mindedness as a virtue

It is unusual to find open-mindedness listed as a virtue in its own right although it would seem to be a tradition in science that intellectual integrity requires an open-mind (see, for example, Hare 2003; Williams 2002). Where the idea of open-mindedness as a virtue does gain support it tends to be categorised as a virtue of the intellect rather than as a virtue of character. It might be assumed that because being open-minded requires the use of cognition then if it is a virtue at all it is a virtue limited to the intellectual domain. The distinction between virtues of the intellect and virtues of the character (sometimes stated as a distinction between the intellectual and the moral virtues) comes from Aristotle. As a result of this distinction there has been a tendency to assume that the realm of action is the province of the moral rather than the intellectual virtues. While assumptions of this kind are understandable in the light of such a distinction it provides only a partial reconstruction of Aristotle's account of the role of the virtues in the life of an individual. For Aristotle, virtues cannot be separated from actions and in this intellectual virtues are no different. Indeed, the virtues of the intellect help to guide us towards right actions and in describing *phronesis* (practical wisdom) Aristotle provides us with an illustration of the close relationship between the virtues of the intellect and the virtues of the character. In this respect open-mindedness is no different. To consider open-mindedness as a virtue is to recognise its place in guiding the actions of a person. This is to say that an account of open-mindedness as a virtue requires that the interdependency between cognition and action be recognised. In this chapter I provide an outline of what is meant by open-mindedness in general and as a virtue in particular; as well as an explanation of why it is a necessary virtue for the practice of nursing.

The nature of open-mindedness

According to Gardner it is a common understanding to say that 'being open-minded about something rules out commitment or belief' (Gardner 1993, p.40). However it is neither clear that this is indeed the commonly held view of open-mindedness nor is it clear that any particular individual would think this to be what is meant by being open-minded. If I were to say that I have an open mind about something it would be possible for a listener to interpret my claim in one of (at least) two ways. They might think, for example, that I have not yet made up my mind or they might think that I am open to being persuaded to change my mind about whatever it is that I am claiming to have an open mind about (other possible interpretations might suggest themselves depending on the context in which the claim to be open-minded is made). Not only is there a clear difference in these two interpretations (the former implies I have not yet come to hold a view, the latter suggests a view has already been formed) but also both of the interpretations appear to be equally valid as everyday understandings of what it means to be open-minded. In both cases it would be true to the general everyday sense of the term that my mind remains open rather than closed about this particular thing. This is to say that I do not have a fixed and unalterable opinion, view or belief about the matter. There may be some things about which I do indeed have a fixed (and perhaps permanent) opinion, view or belief but when I claim to have an open mind about a particular thing I am stating that *in this case* I have an open rather than a closed mind. And there is nothing in what has been said so far that makes one meaning of open-mindedness more correct than the other.

Gardner has a number of concerns related to his claim that to be open-minded is to have not come to hold a belief. He takes this to mean that someone who is open-minded about everything (that is, generally open-minded) cannot at the same time hold any firm beliefs. And, importantly, he claims that one consequence of this for education is: 'the recommendation that we teach children to be open-minded leads to the prescription that we avoid ways of teaching that will promote firm beliefs and that we teach children that it is wrong to have firm beliefs' (p.40). He recognises the desirability of being open-minded about some things but claims that there are just too many things one cannot and should not be open-minded about. Of course it is correct to say that there are limits to open-mindedness and more will be said about this in due course but for now it is worth noting that Gardner's view may be criticised as offering a false dichotomy. That is, it takes as necessary a binary approach to classification or, to put this another way, it takes an 'if something is not an *x* then it must be a *y*' view of open-mindedness. While phrasing questions in this binary fashion is appropriate for some forms of classification it is not appropriate for others. It tends to polarise opinion and can lead to the development of impoverished accounts of phenomena. Gardner's claim that it is not possible to be generally open-minded and at the same time to hold firm beliefs is an inappropriate binary classification that leads him to hold a limited view of the nature of open-mindedness.

The following example illustrates one of the limitations of Gardner's account. It might be that I think it important that I should come to a view on the conditions under which prisoners are held in Camp X-ray at Guantanamo Bay. While I may have a firm view about the sorts of conditions that should be in place in general for those held against their will I can at the same time remain open-minded about whether or not the conditions in which those currently held in Camp X-ray are being kept are acceptable. Thus I may be committed to a view *in general* but not necessarily committed to a view *in particular* (at least in this example).

For the purpose of illustration I might say that my view *in general* is that persons in captivity should not have their autonomy overridden beyond that which is a necessary component of a prison sentence. Thus while an individual may be locked in a prison cell their movements within that cell should not be restricted beyond ensuring their own safety and the safety of others. To tie a prisoner to the bed in her or his cell is to exceed any otherwise legitimate restrictions on her or his autonomy of action. Or to put this another way, while there are legitimate restrictions on the autonomy of action of those in captivity (that is, after all, what it means to be a prisoner) there are nevertheless limits to those restrictions. Furthermore, restrictions to autonomy of thought and restrictions to autonomy of the will are not usually considered to be a legitimate part of captivity.

This means that as a prisoner I would expect that certain autonomous choices remain open to me: choices in relation to worship, exercise, sleep, having milk in my coffee and so on are choices that I must continue to enjoy should I be required to endure any periods of legitimate captivity. And I expect these sorts of choices to be available to others held against their will.

However, my view *in particular*, that is my view about the *particular* conditions in which *particular* persons are being held in a *particular* prison will be a view that requires me to have access to certain sorts of information; information that provides evidence against which I judge whether or not conditions in the particular case meet my view in general of what is acceptable in holding persons against their will. Therefore it remains possible, at least in this instance, for me to remain open-minded in the particular without compromising my strongly held firm general belief. In addition, and despite this separation of the general and particular, I can still remain open-minded about my general firmly held belief in how things ought to be for those held in captivity.

It is likely that Gardner would object to this characterisation of the difference between holding a firm belief in general while being open-minded in particular in the case illustrated above. He might claim that the example supports his own view of what it is to be open-minded precisely because the example offers both something very specific about which to be open-minded (that is where I have not yet come to a view) and a firmly held belief. This is not, he might say, an example of being open-minded about a firmly held belief. And in this he would be partly correct. Yet while it would be tempting to think that because I hold a firm view in general I no longer have an open mind about that firm view this would be to confuse two aspects of open-mindedness. And, if I have understood the literature on open-mindedness correctly, it is these two aspects that are central to the debates between Gardner on the one hand and Hare and McLaughlin on the other.

As already noted, Gardner claims that it is not possible to be open-minded and hold a firm view about the same thing at the same time. He puts this most forcefully when he asks if it is possible for the Pope to be open-minded about the existence of God (Gardner 1993). This is a rhetorical question, for Gardner takes it as absurd that one can be open-minded about a commitment of this nature. Gardner makes a distinction that I interpret as a difference between 'having an open-mind' in the particular (which he claims is the everyday meaning of open-mindedness) and 'being open-minded' in general (which he takes to be inconsistent with holding any firm views at all). Hare and McLaughlin (1994) claim that Gardner's position illustrates a common misunderstanding about the nature of open-mindedness. William Hare puts it thus: 'the open-minded person is one who is able and willing to form an opinion, or revise it, in the light of evidence and argument' (Hare 1988, p.123).

Four categories of open-mindedness

Following this definition I take it that it is possible to be open-minded in four different sorts of ways.

1. I HAVE INSUFFICIENT EVIDENCE ON WHICH TO FORM A FIRM VIEW

This is the position in respect of my view of whether or not those incarcerated in Camp X-ray are being treated appropriately. I have an open mind on this question and remain uncommitted to a *particular* view while maintaining my view *in general*.

2. I HAVE NOT YET GIVEN ATTENTION TO THE MATTER SO I HAVE NO FIRM VIEW

Here I am unable to hold a firm view based on evidence as I have not considered it necessary to come to a firm view, and unless I can be convinced of a need to hold a firm view on the matter I will continue to remain open-minded about it. This is not say that I have no opinion on the matter, but it is to say that my opinion is likely to be based on something other than sufficient evidence or argument.

3. I HAVE GIVEN ATTENTION TO THE MATTER BUT THE INFORMATION IS SUCH THAT I CANNOT ARRIVE AT A FIRM VIEW BASED ON EVIDENCE

This is similar to position 1 above where I remain of the opinion that sufficient information exists and that I anticipate access to that information. In position 3 I have accessed the available information and find the evidence to be inconclusive (the jury is still out, so to speak). It is possible that one day there may be additional and perhaps compelling evidence to enable me to come to a firm view but while this might seem a reasonable expectation in some cases it may be that there are other instances where the evidence is set to remain contestable. As such I remain open to the possibility that any firm view I might have about the matter will be one based on something other than compelling evidence and furthermore will be held with a recognition that there is little, if any, possibility of resolution by evidence or argument.

4. I HAVE GIVEN ATTENTION TO THE MATTER AND THE INFORMATION IS SUCH THAT I CAN COME TO A FIRM VIEW, BUT AT THE SAME TIME I ACCEPT THAT THERE MAY BE A NEED TO RETURN TO 3 ABOVE FROM TIME TO TIME IN THE LIGHT OF NEW EVIDENCE

Here I have come to hold a firm view based on evidence and/or argument, that is to say I am committed to a firm view. For example, if I firmly believe, based on what I perceive to be a set of convincing arguments, that prisoners should be treated in the way outlined earlier,

I will also be committed to the possibility that this firm belief might be wrong. I therefore remain committed to the possibility that, at some future time, I might be presented with an argument or with some evidence that would convince me that I am (was) wrong to hold this particular belief.

It should be noted that this taxonomy is not an attempt to categorise how people come to hold firm beliefs in general, rather it is presented to illustrate four different but legitimate and everyday meanings of open-mindedness. It is clear that individuals do come to hold firm beliefs for many different sorts of reasons only some of which relate to what has been said so far about open-mindedness.

Hare's definition seems to encompass each of these four possibilities and I take it that to be open-minded in this way is a requirement for autonomy. Thus it is possible to hold a firm belief while at the same time remain open to the possibility that that firm belief may subsequently be in need of revision.

Being open-minded

So if I am to be open-minded I can be both committed to a view but open to the possibility that I may be wrong, that is open to revising my firmly held views on the basis of evidence and/or argument. It should not be forgotten that Hare's definition includes the forming as well as the revising of opinion. Thus it includes what might be described as having an open mind (1–3 above) as well as being open-minded (4 above). If I am to claim to be generally open-minded then it would seem to be important that I am not only minded to revise my firmly held beliefs but also that I will not form beliefs without the benefit of the appropriate sorts of evidence and/or argument.

For Gardner being generally open-minded is untenable as he would take this to be to hold no firm beliefs at all but as Hare (1985) points out this is to make the mistake of confusing being generally open-minded with being generally uncommitted. There are many reasons why an individual might be generally uncommitted including the possibility that it may reflect a person's disinclination to engage with issues rather than any inclination to be open-minded. It is true that there are many things about which individuals should remain open-minded in the sense of 1–3 above and hence have no firm beliefs (or at least none based on evidence). But there is also a need for those same individuals to be able to recognise those things about which they should have firm beliefs while at the same time remain open-minded in the sense of 4 above.

To hold no firm beliefs would be to risk unsuccessful navigation in the world and to increase one's vulnerability. Everyday experience suggests that some firmly held beliefs not only protect us from harm (for example, a belief in the damage a motor vehicle can inflict on a pedestrian) but also must be taken to be true if we are to accept that we live in a physical and knowable world.

Two failures of open-mindedness

Following Aristotle I will claim that there are two failures (vices) of open-mindedness. One failure is easy to identify as narrow- or closed-mindedness. Often considered to be the opposite of the open-minded individual, the narrow- or closed-minded person is one who will come to, or hold, a firm view in spite of evidence to the contrary; it describes someone who is closed to the possibility that she or he may be wrong. The other failure is perhaps less obvious and might be described as a failure of the critical component of open-mindedness; that is a tendency to form, or revise, an opinion *without* the benefit of evidence or argument. Such a readiness to believe on weak or insufficient grounds is credulousness. Thus open-mindedness can be described as a virtue lying at a mean between closed-mindedness and credulousness.

While the traditional enemy of open-mindedness is closed-mindedness it is possible that credulousness is a more insidious vice. The closed-minded person will turn away from reasoned argument, will be unprepared to review the evidence and will resist change because they see no reason why that which they currently believe should not continue to serve them well. In contrast the credulous individual will be ever ready to adopt the latest idea without thinking through the evidence or argument on which the proposed change is based or without considering the implications and/or likely consequences of the change.

Closed-mindedness

There are numerous historical examples where evidence that we now take to be compelling was rejected because it did not correspond with the firmly held beliefs of the day. Theories that have come to be recognised as valid but which contradicted the received wisdom of the time have often been ridiculed before gaining general acceptance; their authors subjected to lampooning by both the populace and the eminent. Examples would include: beliefs about the need to exclude women from activities that were believed to be the province of men, activities ranging from voting and medical training to riding bicycles; beliefs about the position of the earth in relation to the universe; and beliefs about the relationship (or lack thereof) between hygiene and infection. These are but three examples of what we now take to be false beliefs. While it may be comforting to note that these examples are from a past in which we imagine people to have been generally less open-minded than we are now, it would be arrogant indeed to believe that we are immune from such closed-minded thinking. For it is possible that some of the firmly held general beliefs we hold in our present era will be similarly derided in a not very distant future. As Williams (2002) points out, we cannot give attention to every crackpot idea that is presented for that would paralyse serious enquiry. Thus it would seem inevitable that some of the ideas that later come to be accepted will have been dismissed inappropriately on the way.

Credulousness

However, there are many who remain ready and willing to support unusual or unorthodox ideas regardless of how fantastic or weird they may appear; indeed, there are those who seem intent on championing seriously wacky ideas as a matter of principle. Such persons are often guilty of credulousness although there may yet be a fine line between the credulous and the visionary. For, as implied in the previous paragraph, it is true that some of the ideas and beliefs we currently cherish will have appeared as just plain crazy to our predecessors. Nevertheless, it is generally the case that the more bizarre an idea appears in relation to the accepted common beliefs of the day the less likely that idea will be taken seriously except by those with credulous tendencies. Of course, this gives us a serious problem if we are to remain open-minded for it seems we need some way of assessing the legitimacy of all evidence and argument before we can come to a view about anything.

Aiming for open-mindedness

Honest enquiry[17] requires open-mindedness and this is the case regardless of whether or not open-mindedness is considered as a virtue. As a virtue, of course, open-mindedness is a disposition rather than some form of obligation; having the virtue one is inclined rather than disinclined to be open-minded. The necessity of being able to know whether or not one should attend to or reject specific evidence or argument is of pressing concern if we are to avoid either of the two failures of open-mindedness outlined above. Although he does not express it in this way, this difficulty does seem to be part of the problem to which Gardner alerts us. In Aristotelian terms it is the problem of hitting the mean in pursuit of the virtue of open-mindedness. In aiming for open-mindedness we aim to avoid the vices of both closed-mindedness and credulousness. This is never going to be an easy task as the history of science tells us for the acceptance of novel ideas is often made more difficult by entrenched positions held by powerful or influential persons or institutions.[18] And in the so-called information age, when information is both freely available and of an almost infinite amount, this problem of assessing the legitimacy of evidence is exponentially more difficult.

Bernard Williams points out that when there is so much information, and when so much of it comes to us from unregulated sources, there is a pressing need for those who wish to make informed judgements about the validity of information to acquire some very specific searching and retrieval skills, as well as the need to engage in what he calls 'processes that are truth-acquiring...such things as careful argument, attention to empirical inquiry, sifting of evidence, and so on' (Williams 2002, p.214). Those who do not know how to sort the wheat from the chaff will forever be at the mercy of their own arbitrary choices of information sources and consequently are very likely to fall into the traps of either closed-mindedness or credulousness, or both. For Williams, the university remains our best chance of avoiding these two vices, but only for as long as the university can remain true to the goals of honest enquiry.

If we aim to be dispositionally open-minded then it is to be supposed that we must remain open-minded about the possibility that what we count as evidence should be extended to include things we would ordinarily reject as legitimate evidence while at the same remaining aware of the possibility that we may be failing in open-mindedness by becoming credulous. One problem here is that for any firmly held belief I have it might be difficult to conceive of the nature of contrary evidence or argument. If it is true that I am unable to imagine what sort of evidence might convince me that I am wrong in one or more of my firmly held beliefs then I am in danger of not being able to recognise the evidence should it be presented. This suggests that being generally open-minded requires the use of imagination and no small amount of intellectual creativity. To aim for open-mindedness is to strive to avoid dismissing evidence to which one should attend and to dismiss evidence that one should avoid. As a minimum this requires sufficient self-awareness about the extent to which one understands the limitations of existing criteria for assessing the value of evidence.

Limits to open-mindedness

Being open-minded about firmly held and fundamental beliefs is problematic and suggests that there are indeed legitimate limitations to open-mindedness. The problem is not so much the idea that there are some things about which we should not ordinarily be open-minded rather it is the question of how we are to know which things fit into this category. This is an example of one of the difficulties of liberalism where an idea has the potential to collapse into itself when confronted with the need to set limits to its own tolerance. If we are to be open-minded then any criteria we use to establish the *things that we should not ordinarily be open-minded about* must not be illiberal criteria, for that would be inconsistent with the idea of open-mindedness in general. The criteria must be such that open-mindedness is encouraged rather than discouraged at least insofar as it promotes human flourishing. As such the criteria cannot be reduced to mere procedural rules for apart from the problem of infinite regress there will remain a need for the exercise of judgement in situations that challenge the normal everyday limitations on open-mindedness. Judgement will also be required because of the need to remain open-minded about the criteria themselves. Any criteria set will inevitably reflect human values and biases and this will require us to remain aware of the possibility that our criteria might act to reduce rather than promote the capacity for human flourishing. Such judgement requires the exercise of those human capacities that afford us the ability to make reasoned judgements and is characterised by Aristotle as practical wisdom.

Even so there is nothing in the fact that I hold firm beliefs about things that fit into the category of *things about which I should not ordinarily be open-minded* that prevents me from remaining open-minded about them in the sense that there may, on occasion, be good reason for calling them into question. As it happens, I am confident that I shall not need to revise many, if any, of these types of firmly held beliefs but I am still open to the possibility that I may be wrong. Practical wisdom may help me to determine those things about which I should hold firm beliefs, while still being open-minded (sense 4 above), if I am to flourish in the world: and it will also help me to recognise those things about which I should remain open-minded in the sense of 1–3 above. The uncertainty about these things reflects our human vulnerability and attempts such as those of Gardner to eliminate this uncertainty by creating clear 'either/or' categories only serve to distract us from one of the inherent difficulties of the human condition.

As noted above, there are legitimate limits to open-mindedness. Gardner (1993) maintains that there is a whole range of issues about which it would be absurd to remain open-minded. Thus, the Pope cannot be open-minded about the existence of God and we should not be open-minded about the wickedness of child abuse. Hare and McLaughlin (1994) accept that there are indeed limits to open-mindedness but, for reasons similar to those outlined above, they do not believe this to undermine their account of open-mindedness. It does, however, cause some difficulties. They note four such limitations which might be categorised as: the practical limit, the rational limit, the moral limit and the logical limit.

1. The practical limit
The practical limit is illustrated by noting that a defendant in a murder trial who is actually innocent would be unwise to be open-minded about his innocence (Hare 1985).

2. The rational limit
The rational limit is the set of firmly held beliefs that it would be bizarre and misleading to claim to be open-minded about. It would only be in very particular and unusual (that is non-everyday) circumstances that doubts would even be entertained. By way of example they suggest that when doing philosophy one might be prepared to be open-minded

about the sorts of things that 'are so basic and fundamental that they must hold if *anything* is ever going to count as evidence' (Hare and McLaughlin 1994, p.242; original emphasis).

3. The moral limit
Hare and McLaughlin are more tentative about the nature and scope of the moral limit but they do say 'There may also be beliefs...of morality which are so fundamental to our understanding of what morality is that we cannot make sense of the suggestion that they may be false' (p.242).

4. The logical limit
The logical limit is set by the terms in which open-mindedness is understood. Thus it is not possible to be open-minded about open-mindedness itself because to attempt to be open-minded about open-mindedness is to demonstrate a commitment to open-mindedness.

Bramall's critique
It is at this point that Bramall takes issue with the terms within which the debate is conducted. Bramall claims that to be open-minded and to accept the logical limitation is to accept and be committed to a liberal rational methodology without being open-minded about that methodology (or, possibly, even without recognising the adherence to a particular methodology). The liberal rational account is, Bramall maintains, a product of the Enlightenment project that fails to recognise, or is perhaps unable to recognise, its own perspective as prejudiced. Drawing upon hermeneutic phenomenology Bramall concludes that: 'Our view of the world is...always constrained by our conceptual horizons. All understanding is always one interpretation of phenomena that could be interpreted differently from different categorical and conceptual frameworks' (Bramall 2000, p.207). In arguing for 'something like a virtue of hermeneutic open-mindedness' (p.209) he claims that the logical limitation of open-mindedness as conceived in the liberal rational tradition can be overcome. Hermeneutic open-mindedness allows for 'the possibility for individuals to be open-minded about all their important beliefs including the commitment to open-mindedness itself' (p.211).

As an alternative, Bramall suggests the need for a disposition to be not only open-minded in terms of rational evidence and argument as put forward by Hare but also to be open-minded about our own worldview. The essential difference being that not only will I be 'able and willing to form an opinion, or revise it, in the light of evidence and argument' but that I will also be able and willing to extend the scope of my evidence and argument by using frames of reference hitherto alien to my firmly held perspective of the world. If I understand Bramall correctly he is asking us to extend our view to take account of evidence and argument that we would normally reject on rational liberal grounds; that is, evidence and/or argument that does not meet the usual rational liberal criteria employed to provide legitimacy. While I can appreciate that this is indeed consistent with the notion of open-mindedness, particularly as proposed by Bramall, I remain concerned about how we are to know what is to count and what is not to count as appropriate evidence and/or argument. This is a pressing problem for nurses if they are to avoid being accused of credulousness. The idea of open-mindedness as a virtue is strong in Bramall's account. He talks of the 'dispositionally anti-dogmatic' person who seems to be the main purpose of educating for open-mindedness. The challenge for educators, of course, is to create an environment in which open-mindedness can flourish and this will be discussed further in Chapter 6.

Why open-mindedness is necessary for nursing practice

One of my firmly held beliefs is that nursing is a MacIntyrean practice (Sellman 2000, 2010) engagement with which requires what MacIntyre (1985) describes as the three core virtues of a practice: the virtues of honesty, courage and justice. In the previous chapter I presented a case for accepting trustworthiness as one additional necessary professional virtue. In this chapter I claim that open-mindedness is a second additional necessary professional virtue for the practice of nursing.

There is an emphasis in nursing, as there is in other social professions, for practice to be based on evidence. The major assumption behind this is that practice based on evidence is more likely to be beneficial to those whose interests the profession is designed to serve. A further assumption is that individual practitioners have the capacity or willingness to change their practice in the light of appropriate sorts of evidence. If this is true, and assuming that individuals will only change their practice if they believe there to be benefit in doing so, then not only is it necessary for individual practitioners to be disposed to change their practice but it is also necessary for them to form and/or revise their (related to practice) beliefs on the basis of evidence and/or argument. This is to say that if nurses are to base their practice on evidence then they must be dispositionally open-minded. It follows that those nurses who are not dispositionally open-minded (that is do not have the virtue of open-mindedness) are failing in some way.

Walsh and Ford (1989) provide many examples of nursing practices where rituals continue despite a wealth of (research) evidence that demonstrates the lack of an evidence base for those practices and offers recommendations for evidence-based practice. This contributes to, and perhaps is even explanatory of, the 'practice-theory' gap. Students of nursing often complain of the discrepancy between what they are taught in the classroom and what they see practised in the clinical areas. Manual handling provides a telling example.

In the UK it was once the case that nurses were required to lift patients. During the 1970s an early attempt to utilise evidence as a basis for practice led to a move to adopt lifting techniques using the principles of ergonomics and correct positioning to minimise the potential for harm to patients and/or staff. The impetus for introducing the idea of 'safe lifting' came from a recognition of the high numbers of nurses lost to the profession as a result of back injury. Despite the best efforts of health authorities in providing training in safe lifting there was a marked reluctance by clinical nurses to change the traditional approach of lifting (particularly the 'underarm' lift) despite widespread acceptance of evidence demonstrating the potential hazards to both patients and staff.

Some of the techniques designed to avoid harm were adopted during the 1980s only to be subsequently discredited by new evidence. In addition, European directives led to the introduction of restrictions on permissible lifting loads which has effectively outlawed the lifting of adult patients. Hence, the term manual handling rather than lifting. There are a number of devices designed to make easy and effortless the manual handling of patients, many of which are inexpensive, readily available and relatively simple to use: yet resistance to the use of these devices is apparent to any who work in clinical areas. And worse still discredited lifting techniques, including the 'underarm' lift, continue.

In order to avoid being accused of professional misconduct a nurse must be sure that the procedures and practices she or he undertakes are compatible with current best practice. That is, practices which a body of contemporary professionals would consider to be consistent with practice based on the best current and generally available evidence. This does not need to be evidence at the cutting edge (as it were) but it does need to be practice based on valid conclusions drawn from the best currently and generally available evidence; conclusions, furthermore, that it would be reasonable for any competent practitioner to recognise as valid. This together with the professional requirement for a registered nurse to maintain her or his professional competence and the moral requirement to protect patients from harm makes it necessary for each practitioner to identify and abandon any unsafe practices.

Measured thus a nurse who routinely continues to lift rather than manually handle is failing to practise in a way that is consistent with current best evidence-based practice. While it is important to retain an open-mind insofar as it is possible that new evidence may become available to show that current manual handling techniques are not best practice it is folly to suggest that (under normal circumstances) the current evidence implies anything other than nurses should manually handle rather than lift.

Closed-mindedness would seem to be a major factor in situation in which nurses continue to lift in spite of overwhelming evidence demonstrating the potential for harm. This can be categorised as a type 1 risk of harm (the sort of risk that can be substantially reduced by one's own actions; see Chapter 2) and yet the failure by many to take preventative and protective action continues. Those who lift know they should not and the most common reason cited is a lack of time. There are indeed local obstacles to safe manual handling including: a lack of easily available equipment; equipment that is perceived as complicated and time consuming to use; insufficient training in the proper use of equipment particularly where training does not keep up with changes in personnel, and so on. But these obstacles only remain as obstacles in the face of resistance to changes in practice. It suggests that nurses who continue to lift when there is such a weight of evidence (and it should be emphasised here that there is no controversy about the compelling nature of this evidence) is a failure of open-mindedness. As Aristotle reminds us in the *Nichomachean Ethics* (1953) a virtue is a disposition to act. When I claim that open-mindedness is a virtue I am claiming something more than just the forming or revising of beliefs; I am claiming that the open-minded nurse is one who is disposed to act in a manner consistent with those beliefs. So it is not that I am claiming nurses should revise only their beliefs but that they should also act in a way that is consistent with their beliefs, particularly where a failure to do so may put themselves or others at risk of harm. And if one of the legitimate aims of nursing is human flourishing, as suggested throughout this book, then a failure to protect patients from an avoidable risk of harm is a failure in professional practice.

So while (because of the weight of evidence against lifting in general) an open-minded nurse is committed to a firm view about the undesirability of lifting adult patients this does not mean that she or he will never resort to lifting even when she or he knows that the potential for harm from lifting exists. It may be that in an emergency such as a fire, a nurse may believe it necessary to lift if the equipment cannot be set up in time.[19] For a nurse (while still recognising manual handling is normally appropriate) to lift in this sort of case is to demonstrate open- rather than closed-mindedness about lifting. That is to say that while the nurse may have a suitably firm view that lifting is generally inappropriate, that firm view can remain open to revision in a particular situation where in her or his opinion complying with the general injunction not to lift may have more harmful consequences than lifting. Of course, decisions of this nature cannot be mere arbitrary decisions rather they require the application of what I have termed *professional phronesis* (Sellman 2009).

This example of the general inappropriateness of lifting is in sharp contrast to the wholesale adoption of advocacy as a legitimate part of the role of the nurse during the 1980s and 1990s with very little critical debate, and certainly without a universally accepted definition of the term. Seedhouse (2000) reviewed the ways in which advocacy had been interpreted by nursing scholars and finds disagreement and variation together with a lack of any clear analysis of the concept as it relates to practising nurses. This I take to be a different sort of failure of open-mindedness; a tendency to form a belief on the basis of insufficient evidence and/or argument, that is, credulousness. It is tempting to think that it might be case that nurses are able to quickly make up their minds on the basis of the available evidence (after all nurses are often required to make clinical decisions rapidly) but this would be to mistake credulousness for open-mindedness. Advocacy was adopted as one of the 'big ideas' of its time and it has become part of the received wisdom of nursing.

Limits to open-mindedness in nursing practice

All that has been said so far about the importance of open-mindedness for nursing practice has been said in recognition that one legitimate end of nursing practice is human flourishing, in particular the flourishing of *more-than-ordinarily* vulnerable persons. And because some beliefs and actions are inconsistent with human flourishing this puts some additional legitimate limits on open-mindedness for nursing practice. On this account any nursing actions that interfere with human flourishing are actions that nurses should not perform. For example, the routine killing of patients is prohibited not only because it is against the law and contrary to the standards of the profession but also, and perhaps more importantly, because it is inconsistent with the general concept of human flourishing.

As outlined earlier a general disposition towards open-mindedness brings with it some difficulties for everybody. The everyday experience of those working in health care is such that it brings nurses and other health care workers closer to the margins of the limitations of open-mindedness in very practical ways. Nurses are often confronted with situations that challenge ordinary everyday assumptions about issues taken as largely unproblematic by the general populace. This generates something of a problem as there would seem to be a greater tension for nurses between the idea of a general disposition towards open-mindedness on the one hand and the challenges to *those things which we should not ordinarily be open-minded about* on the other. This is to say that there are some things about which is it especially important nurses should hold firm beliefs for the absence of such beliefs would, except, perhaps, in some extreme and exceptional circumstances, be unprofessional and contrary to human flourishing. Some of the *things nurses should not ordinarily be open-minded about* are considered below.

In common with human activity in general, working as a nurse presupposes a set of firmly held beliefs in the existence of a physical and knowable world. It presupposes the physical reality inter alia of patients and nurses, of buildings and medicines, of human life, healing, and death and so on. Without these kinds of firmly held beliefs there would be little point in the activity of nursing. The certainties we feel about such things suggests that these are not the sorts of things that we should normally be open-minded about, for if we entertained doubts about these things we would surely become lost in a haze of perpetual uncertainty and cease to act altogether. These types of firmly held beliefs are part of the practical limitations of open-mindedness.

The particular beliefs that *nurses should not ordinarily be open-minded about* that need to be considered here are those that might be categorised as those belonging to the moral domain. McLaughlin provides a forceful argument that there are some aspects of the moral domain that are so basic and fundamental that it does not make sense (at least in ordinary circumstances) to call them into question. He says:

> The sorts of moral sensitivities, beliefs, judgements and commitments which have been mentioned are basic or fundamental to the moral domain itself and to call them into question, or to be disposed to do so, might be considered to undermine the moral domain itself and to put the questioner outside that domain. (McLaughlin 2003b, p.23)

The idea that nurses should be open-minded about centrally important concerns such as the need to demonstrate a caring attitude towards patients and about working towards the relief of suffering seems inappropriate.[20] As does the idea that nursing has nothing to do with enabling the flourishing of *more-than-ordinarily* vulnerable persons. It does seem that to be open-minded about questions of this nature is antithetical to nursing as a practice and questions of this sort do appear to be candidates for inclusion in the *things that nurses should not be open-minded about* category.

Aiming for open-mindedness in the practice of nursing

Some of the difficulties involved in aiming for open-mindedness in general have been discussed earlier in this chapter. The main difficulty is the Aristotelian problem of hitting the mean and as Williams suggests there are a number of intellectual skills that can be usefully brought to bear on the problem. The intellectual skills of analysis, synthesis and evaluation will assist individuals to determine the legitimacy of evidence and argument. In a practical activity such as nursing the importance of knowing which evidence to attend to becomes ever more pressing precisely because the flourishing of *more-than-ordinarily* vulnerable persons is at stake. Additionally, assessing the value of evidence and argument on which to base trustworthy practice also requires those very virtues that MacIntyre identifies as constitutive of the practice itself. Thus, being open-minded requires the virtues of honesty, justice and courage. The nurse who is disposed to honesty, justice and courage is more likely to be inclined to recognise the limitations of the evidence base for practice; is more likely to engage in critical review of evidence and is more likely to continue to seek out evidence in the pursuit of best practice. Such a nurse approximates what I have termed an honest enquirer who, as Haack puts it:

> wants the true answer to his question: if he is inquiring into whether cigarette smoking causes cancer, he wants to end up believing that cigarette smoking causes cancer if cigarette smoking causes cancer, and that it doesn't if it doesn't (and that it's a lot more complicated than that if it's a lot more complicated than that). (Haack 1998, p.9)

In short, such a nurse genuinely wants to know whether her or his practice is contributing to the flourishing of *more-than-ordinarily* vulnerable persons and in pursuit of this goal is open to the possibility that current practice may need to change in the light of appropriate evidence. Thus this nurse is open-minded and trustworthy for she or he is taking seriously her or his epistemic responsibilities. As such, this idealised nurse will be demonstrating what I termed in Chapter 1 *professional phronesis*, that is, a practical wisdom born out of engaging with nursing as a MacIntyrean practice in a trustworthy and open-minded way.

Evidence and open-mindedness for nursing practice

I have noted that aiming for open-mindedness requires inter alia making an effort to assess the legitimacy of evidence in order to attend to the sorts of evidence necessary for the pursuit of nursing as a MacIntyrean practice. In Chapter 3 I noted that ideas about the nature of nursing remain contested and it is, therefore, important for nurses to be in a position to assess the evidence on which competing ideas rely. After all, any serious appeal to evidence must anticipate appropriate challenges to that evidence. Evidence provides one means by which we can make informed choices about the appropriateness of nursing interventions. But it is possible that we can easily be misled about legitimacy of evidence if we do not pay attention to the way in which evidence becomes available. In his discussion about the marketplace of ideas, Bernard Williams (2002) notes that there is a very real danger that the unregulated marketplace that is the Internet while making information freely available to all those with a computer and with world wide web access also provides opportunities for those with particular sets of ideas to keep those ideas isolated from truth-acquiring processes. As such then the Internet poses a particularly insidious threat to honest enquiry. In addition, there is a tendency within nursing for authority to be invested in the journals in which evidence is published. This leads to a general perception that if something is published in a journal afforded a high status, or with a high impact factor it has a higher 'truth' value than if it were published in journal of lower status or with a lower impact factor score. Thus the findings of enquiries can gain status as somehow *more truthful* or *more compelling* when they are published in one journal rather than another. And if this becomes part of a received wisdom of the profession then the temptation to think 'if it has been published in journal x it must be right' may be irresistible to both the closed-minded and the credulous nurse. Additionally, it matters not how much protestation is made by the authors of papers in these publications that their findings should be treated with caution because of design flaws or other noted weaknesses. In published nursing research there remains a tendency for authors to couch their conclusions and recommendations in terms that suggest the acknowledged limitations are not really that important after all, rather what is important is, for example, that their findings are consistent with the findings of (most) other studies in the subject area. And further, there is a tendency for the consumers of nursing research to pay attention to findings in ways that might be best described as credulous (that is, the tendency to adopt a belief on insufficient grounds).

Evidence is indeed a necessary component of how we should come to believe the veracity or otherwise of assertions but it is possible that few individuals exercise open-mindedness in forming beliefs. It may be that rather than using evidence to form our beliefs, some use evidence to support existing beliefs. This is not to say that we cannot form beliefs on the basis of evidence nor it is to say that our beliefs cannot be revised in the light of evidence but it is to say that there may be an understandable tendency to choose our evidence to suit our beliefs. A stronger version of this is developed by MacIntyre and expressed in his claim that our moral choices may ultimately all be arbitrary. By way of example, when asked why we think *x* is a good we might reply that *x* is a good because, following utilitarian reasoning, *x* meets the criterion for goodness; but when asked why we should accept utilitarian reasoning we would surely struggle to say anything more than utilitarian reasoning seems to offer useful criteria by which to determine the good. Evidence to support a firmly held belief such as a belief in the value of utilitarian reasoning may be available but it is likely to take the form of a selection of those things that fit; it is likely to be anecdotal; and it is likely to cohere with what we already believe to be the good in any case. In this respect such use of evidence (however this is to be defined) is the same sort of use of evidence that we see at work in conspiracy theory, in tragedy and comedy in literature, and in the thinking of credulous individuals.

Becoming an open-minded nurse

Being open-minded as a nurse is fraught with difficulty especially as much of what nurses do is prescribed by contractual obligations, institutional and hierarchical traditions, nursing codes and various procedures and protocols. These factors give rise to tensions between individual and corporate professional responsibilities. Given these constraints it is clear that there is a need for *professional phronesis* in order that each nurse can negotiate her or his way in pursuit of nursing as a MacIntyrean practice. As both MacIntyre and Potter note there is an additional need for institutional arrangements to be at the very least sympathetic to the idea of virtuous practice if individuals are to be enabled to practice in virtuous ways. And an appropriate institutional stance is one that allows practitioners to exercise discretion.

Many institutions use protocols as a way of attempting to standardise practice but it should be evident that protocols can only ever account for a finite range of possibilities. There will always remain a need for professional discretion and judgement; that is, practical wisdom or what I have termed *professional phronesis*. The dispositionally open-minded nurse will exercise this *professional phronesis* with each new case, even where at first sight a patient would appear to fit into the category the protocol is designed to serve. The open-minded nurse will not only be open-minded about the validity and currency of the protocol in general but also about the appropriateness of the protocol for a given individual patient, that is, open-minded in the particular. Any other position would seem to undermine the notion of an autonomous and accountable practitioner. The closed-minded nurse will either ignore the protocol altogether or be inclined to follow the protocol regardless of its validity and regardless of individual differences among the patients for whom the protocol is designed. The credulous nurse may abandon the protocol on spurious, inadequate or insufficient grounds and in the process render any attempt at systematic care redundant.

By way of a contrast the open-minded nurse will have a number of options in relation to protocols and will need to exercise *professional phronesis* in order to choose from a range of possible courses of action. Thus she or he will need to remain open to a number of possibilities including: the possibility that the protocol may be wrong; the possibility that the protocol may be in need of revision; the possibility that she or he may be wrong to follow the protocol in general; and the possibility that she or he may be wrong to follow the protocol in any particular instance. For to follow a protocol when conditions are such that harm rather than good ensues is not only to pursue a wilful disregard for appropriate profession conduct but it is also to practice with insufficient regard for the flourishing of *more-than-ordinarily* vulnerable persons.

To put this into a practical context, imagine that a patient has a particular type of wound which is of a kind appropriate for a specific treatment protocol where dressing x is required to be renewed daily and is the current accepted best practice for that particular type of wound. It would be reasonable for an individual nurse to start with an assumption that she or he can be relatively secure in the knowledge that this is indeed the best evidence-based practice for that wound but no nurse can continue to use that dressing if other evidence points to a failure of dressing x to aid the healing process in the wound of a particular individual patient. The nurse must be able to deviate from the protocol when the occasion requires but in so doing the nurse needs to be sure that there is sufficient evidence on which to base a decision to deviate. This requires the exercise of *professional phronesis* and represents the essence of autonomous and accountable practice. The nurse is justified in following the established protocol (using dressing x) provided the protocol remains dynamic (that is, is updated to take account of new and compelling evidence). Thus the nurse cannot merely rely on the protocol for if the protocol becomes out of date the nurse who continues to use dressing x in spite of evidence to indicate that it is no longer best practice will be demonstrating inter alia a failure of open-mindedness.

In practice, and in order to avoid being found guilty of professional misconduct, a nurse needs to be confident that the evidence and/ or argument on which she or he bases practice satisfies the test of compliance with a body of contemporary professional opinion. As such there is a sense in which a nurse is right to be wary of using sources of evidence and/or argument that do not already have legitimacy among fellow professionals. Given the pervasive influence of the so-called 'hierarchy of evidence' (Hek, Judd and Moule 2002), the tendency for nurses to seek 'hard' scientific (rather than 'soft' qualitative) evidence for practice is unsurprising. From this perspective the legitimacy test rests on a majority view of what counts as evidence and makes the use of evidence from sources perceived as outside of the mainstream or on the margins of professional respectability problematic. A nurse who uses evidence from sources outside the normal boundaries of this legitimacy test will need to argue the case for its acceptance. The risks (and effort) involved in drawing from sources with uncertain legitimacy may serve to act as a barrier to open-mindedness. For if it is at the cost of risking accusations of unprofessional conduct, then it is difficult to imagine why a nurse would want to choose evidence from anywhere other than 'respectable' or 'sanctioned' sources. This is to say that if the only evidence perceived as legitimate is narrowly conceived as that which results from 'scientific' research then the nurse who uses evidence from sources that do not meet this gold standard will risk censure.

While the closed-minded nurse is unlikely to challenge the boundaries of putative legitimacy, both the open-minded and the credulous nurse may find the restrictions imposed by this hierarchy of evidence difficult. Yet this similarity between the credulous and the open-minded nurse is superficial for while the former will struggle to assess the provenance of information, the latter will endeavour to adopt a critical stance. Thus the open-minded nurse will guard against spurious evidence and/or disingenuous argument. Further, and unlike the credulous nurse, the motivation of the open-minded nurse in seeking to extend the range of evidence for practice will be primarily for the benefit of patients. For these reasons, closed-mindedness seems likely to operate as a force militating against change. Hence, obstacles to becoming dispositionally open-minded are external as well as internal and it looks as though learning to be open-minded requires a certain degree of courage in the face of such forces. Nevertheless, and in spite of these difficulties it still seems that a nurse must strive to become a dispositionally open-minded practitioner if she or he is serious in aiming to enable the flourishing of *more-than-ordinarily* vulnerable persons.

6 The Place of the Virtues in the Education of Nurses

In this book I have begun a preliminary exploration of what it means to understand nursing as a practice in the sense that MacIntyre uses that term. Insofar as conceiving of nursing as a MacIntyrean practice indicates excellence, it provides an idealisation of nursing to which those who wish to be good nurses can aspire in pursuit of the goal of helping *more-than-ordinarily* vulnerable persons to flourish. Evinced in this idealised conception of a nurse is the care and compassion that underpins the enterprise of nursing and those who subscribe to it must aim to cultivate the appropriate virtues: this is to say that those who wish to engage with nursing as a practice will need to cultivate inter alia the three core virtues of honesty, justice and courage as well the professional virtues of trustworthiness and open-mindedness. A good nurse in this conception is one who genuinely wishes to enable the flourishing of *more-than-ordinarily* vulnerable persons. Those who do cultivate the virtues necessary for nursing will characteristically act in ways that promote the flourishing of the patients and at the same time will enhance their own flourishing *qua* humans.

Because nurses work with *more-than-ordinarily* vulnerable persons nursing is an inherently moral practice for (whether they recognise it or not) the actions of nurses will have an impact on patients' flourishing. It follows that the education of nurses is inevitably of a moral kind and it seems desirable that nurse teachers should aim to enable students of nursing to cultivate appropriate civic and professional virtues in order that they may learn to engage with nursing as a practice. While the ideal is that those who engage with nursing as a practice cultivate 'full' virtue it is necessary to recognise that for some (perhaps many) the fragmentation of modernity makes this difficult. Nevertheless, it would seem appropriate to aim, as a minimum, for the cultivation of the very specific professional virtues (of trustworthiness and open-mindedness) tailored to the practice of nursing. Thus one function of nurse teachers is to provide opportunities for students of nursing to come to recognise, understand and develop the specific application and expression of trustworthiness and open-mindedness in nursing practice.

The nature of this moral education in any particular institution will depend upon the assumptions about normative ethics held in that institution. In this book I have accepted what Steutel and Carr (1999) describe as an aretaic virtue ethics as forming the most appropriate grounding for a moral education consistent with the idea of nursing as a practice. Arguing that a broad conception of virtue ethics (and thus a broad conception of a virtue-based moral education) would include Kohlbergian as well as Kantian and utilitarian understandings of virtue, Steutel and Carr define an aretaic virtue ethics as consistent with the general thrust of virtue ethics as contrasted with Kantian and utilitarian ethics in which it is the acts of persons (rather than the persons themselves) that provide the focus for evaluation. It is an aretaic (as opposed to a deontic) ethics because the primary focus is related to 'the evaluation of persons, their characters, intentions and motives' (Steutel and Carr 1999, p.8). Presupposing the existence of character, an aretaic virtue ethics requires that moral judgements include judgements about the virtues that go to make up the character of an individual. Consequently a moral education predicated on an aretaic virtue ethics will be concerned with cultivating the virtues. On this account the moral education of nurses is an education that seeks to encourage the development of those virtues that make possible nursing as a practice in the MacIntyrean sense. This is contrasted with much that is commonplace in higher education in general and in nursing education in particular where the aims of, for example, the teaching of ethics to nurses may be predicated on ideas of the intellectualisation of knowledge separated in some sense from the world of nursing practice. In this chapter I make a preliminary excursion into a discussion about the implications of an aretaic virtue ethics approach to the moral education of nurses.

Nursing education as moral education

In this scheme the essence of education for nursing is the cultivation in nurses of certain sorts of virtues, virtues that are both constitutive of nursing as a practice and of flourishing for nurses *qua* humans. We might refer to these as the virtues of nursing. Cultivating these sorts of virtues inclines students and practitioners towards recognising their own practical learning needs. So, for example, in cultivating trustworthiness the nurse comes to understand that being trustworthy requires that she or he develop the practical skills and competences necessary to practice safe nursing in relation to the patients in her or his care. However, the aim of nurse education as here stated is primarily to enable the flourishing of *more-than-ordinarily* vulnerable persons rather than the flourishing of nurses. Consistent with nursing as a practice in the MacIntyrean sense this requires nurses to develop a unity of virtue at least insofar as these virtues find expression in the practice of nursing. These virtues include in particular the virtues of honesty, courage and justice as well as the professional virtues of trustworthiness and open-mindedness.

Additionally, and consistent with an Aristotelian conception of virtue, is a requirement for the development of what I have termed *professional phronesis* (Sellman 2008, 2009), that is the development of a practical wisdom that is specifically geared towards guiding action in nursing practice. Inherent in these virtues of nursing is a requirement for a general disposition of good will towards particular others; those, that is, who are *more-than-ordinarily* vulnerable. Elsewhere I have noted that this needs to be a good will in a strong rather than weak sense and I have made some suggestions about what good will in a strong sense requires (Sellman 2009). The distinction helps to differentiate between the nurse who is merely well-intentioned (good will in a weak sense) and one who recognises the actions necessary to ensure their good intentions lead to good rather than harm at least insofar as this can ever be determined in advance (good will in the strong sense). So unlike the nurse with a good will in the weak sense, the nurse with a good will in the strong sense knowingly acts in ways that are informed rather than uniformed, skilled rather than unskilled, and consistent rather than inconsistent with the flourishing of *more-than-ordinarily* vulnerable persons.

The nature of moral education

Writing in 1967, Wilson, Williams and Sugarman noted that 'Moral education...is as yet a name for nothing clear' (p.32). Judging from the continuing debates in the literature it is not at all obvious that the nature of moral education is very much clearer now than it was then. However, the argument that Wilson *et al.* emphasise against a conception of moral education as an attempt to get people to act in ways that are consistent with morally acceptable behaviour without taking account of individual moral agency is no longer of central concern. In reflecting the general acceptance that moral education is distinct from moral training, O'Hear writes: 'what we want from moral education is not any sort of adherence to moral principles, but an adherence that is fully internalized and does not require policing' (O'Hear 1998, p.15).

It appears that the (mis)conception of moral education as moral training has been replaced by arguments about the relative merits of what Steutel and Carr describe as a deontic version of moral education on the one hand and an aretaic version on the other. Where the emphasis in the former is placed primarily on judgements about the morality of the actions of agents, the latter highlights the importance of moral character as well as the morality of actions. Noddings and Slote offer a three-way division of approaches to moral education. They say:

> Virtue ethics...would naturally encourage a form of moral education in which schools and parents would seek to inculcate good character in the form of...habitual virtues. Kantian/ Rawlsian rationalism/liberalism would seemingly encourage moral education to take the form of developing certain capacities for moral reasoning and certain very general principles that can be applied to different moral dilemmas...[and] an ethic of care would most naturally see moral education as a matter of children's coming to an intelligent emotional understanding of the good or harmful effects of their actions on the lives of other people... (Noddings and Slote 2003, p.349)

For the purposes of this book the differences in approaches noted by Steutel and Carr on the one hand and by Noddings and Slote on the other are less important than the fact that they both reflect the idea that of central concern in moral education is the debate about the basis from which moral education should proceed. This suggests that distinction between moral education and moral training that Wilson *et al.* believed to be so important is no longer necessary for it has become generally accepted that moral education requires the exercise of moral agency. Nevertheless it is an important distinction that has a direct bearing on the arguments outlined in this book. For this reason the distinction between moral education and moral training will be rehearsed.

Being, or becoming, moral (rather than merely 'acting' in morally acceptably ways) requires the freedom to choose to act in one way rather than another. A person who has been conditioned to act in particular ways not from choice but from, say, indoctrination cannot be considered a fully realised moral agent. So merely attempting to get people to act morally is not moral education as here conceived. Once we recognise that moral education requires moral agency we must recognise that moral education is complex and will require considerable intellectual as well as practical effort on the part of both learner and teacher. Wilson *et al.* argue for moral education as education '...imparting those skills which are necessary to make good or reasonable moral decisions and to act on them' (Wilson *et al.* 1967, p.27) and in so doing they liken moral teaching to the teaching of science as teaching a method rather than the imparting of information; that is, the teaching of science undertaken with an appropriate regard for the traditions and forms of enquiry of the subject. Where the real lesson of science education is to understand the standards of scientific enquiry, to be able to recognise when science is done with integrity, open-mindedness and so on (the internal goods of science in MacIntyre's terms) in a genuine attempt to find out how things really are, the real object of moral education is to enable individuals to express moral agency in the honest pursuit of human good. On this account the ethical nurse is one who genuinely seeks to make and act upon moral decisions that aim for the good of *more-than-ordinarily* vulnerable persons. Making and acting upon genuinely moral decisions requires accepting one's own moral responsibility and doing so on the basis of seeking an understanding of (as Aristotle might say) the universals as well as the particulars of human flourishing in relation not only to the *more-than-ordinarily* vulnerable person with whom one is confronted but also to oneself.

Moral education or moral training?

We have seen that nursing is more that the mere competent completion of tasks for such a description would provide only an impoverished view of an inherently complex activity. Of course it is important that a nurse practice with a minimum of safe competence in whatever particular skills are required given the specific type of nursing work with which she or he is engaged. Developing some of the necessary skills and competences requires training, thus training (as opposed to education in a wider sense) is a component of nurse education. But training someone to carry out a particular activity implies that they must learn to undertake a task or set of tasks following a set of rules of the kind: if x then y. Thus training is involved when someone is taught to insert twelve 5cm bolts into the correct holes in the correct order when working in a factory on an assembly line. And this is perfectly acceptable in terms of learning to undertake a particular task. Once learned it is (in its simplest form) merely a matter of repeating the task on each new widget in the fairly secure knowledge that the next widget to appear will be of the same design, size, shape and so on as the last. Training on this conception is designed to lead to the performance of specific actions in a particular order for an identified purpose.

Of course, patients are not widgets so training for nursing can never be of the same order as illustrated here in this simple sense. There may be training for nursing but this must be limited to competence in performance of tasks in a universal sense. At the extreme this requires an unquestioning response to a particular situation, request or order. In this sense a paratrooper is trained to jump from a plane when a particular command or signal is given and a nurse is trained to give chest compressions during a cardiopulmonary resuscitation attempt. While there may be opportunities when each might wish to question the purpose(s) to which their actions are being put, what the paratrooper and nurse share in these examples is that they are required to do what they have been trained to do when they are required to do it. The paratrooper may be uneasy about the conduct or legality of the mission but, assuming he has been properly trained, will still jump when the order comes, and the nurse may have doubts about the dignity of resuscitating this particular patient (why not let him die in peace?) but will participate as long as the resuscitation attempt continues. And this sort of training is necessary wherever the pursuit of goals requires the collective effort of individuals who must subordinate themselves to the commands of others if specific goals are to be achieved. The paratrooper who refuses to jump will jeopardise the mission not only because he will no longer play his part but also because he will delay the launch of other paratroopers who may then land in the wrong place; the nurse who refuses to begin chest compressions will very likely (if there is no replacement) jeopardise the resuscitation attempt because one other member of the team must take on an additional role.

While we can say that both the paratrooper and the nurse are moral beings, if they so act *only* because of a successful training programme then it is difficult to conclude that they are acting as fully realised moral agents for they are not choosing to act as such, rather they are acting in response to a command. They are being used for some purpose which they may or may not find morally acceptable or defensible, some purpose, moreover, that is not necessarily one they would pursue as independent moral agents. Thus in these circumstances they are merely instrumental in pursuing goals set by others and in one important sense it does not matter whether or not they share those goals. The actions of our paratrooper and nurse might be consistent with moral behaviour but the extent to which they are being moral is, at best, disputable. To act morally is to act intentionally and implies the freedom to choose to act in one rather than in other possible ways. Training of the kind to which our paratrooper and nurse have been subjected seems to compromise moral agency as it is not at all clear that actions born of such training fall into the sphere of freely chosen moral actions. Of course we might say that those whose actions result from mere obedience have failed as moral agents and where such persons allow their actions to be used for unethical purposes we can, and indeed do, hold them accountable for failing to recognise the immorality of those acts. And this forms the basis of legal rulings under which merely 'following orders' does not constitute an acceptable defence. After all, our paratrooper and our nurse are both morally culpable insofar as they are free to refuse to follow orders, and morally speaking we require them to refuse to follow orders that are immoral in terms of means or ends.

Following this line of argument it is tempting to think that training does not have a moral component but this would be to fail to recognise the moral agency inherent in the human capacity to identify 'immoral' orders and to refuse to act in immoral ways (although there are of course situations where individuals might be coerced to comply with immoral commands). Yet the idea of training for moral behaviour or moral training is one fraught with logical and conceptual difficulties. The idea of training people to act in morally acceptable ways is a paradox for it implies a training in obedience and mere unthinking obedience to authority denies the possibility of moral agency. In this sense moral training is a form of indoctrination and as pointed out in Chapter 1, indoctrination is inconsistent with education for citizenship in liberal democracies. It is also inconsistent with an education that purports to enable nurses to use their capacity for independent practical reasoning in the pursuit of safe, competent and ethical care of patients. So insofar as nurses are trained to do certain things training cannot neglect moral agency. Even apparently simple tasks such as measuring blood pressure or transferring a person from bed to chair may take on moral significance in the practice situation. Not only is it possible that a nurse or student may have to choose between measuring one patient's blood pressure and transferring a different patient from bed to chair but the choice may turn out to be of great consequence if for example there are reasons why neither of those tasks ought to be undertaken because of some change in the condition of one or other patient that the nurse or student has failed to observe.

So we might say that while training is a necessary component of nursing education, especially for the development of particular skills and in order to act 'automatically' in certain sorts of situations, that training not only has limited application in terms of being a registered nurse (for health care assistants are often trained in this sense but do not as a result become registered nurses) but also must be undertaken with due regard for the moral implications of the actions for which individuals are being trained. Nurses may not be in a position to refuse to resuscitate a patient (for decisions about whether or not to resuscitate are not normally within a nurse's sphere of authority) but they can, and arguably should, become involved in discussions in which decisions about patients' resuscitation status are made. Just because a nurse is trained and skilled in resuscitation does not mean that she or he should begin a resuscitation attempt on a patient for whom such an attempt is inappropriate. However, a nurse is obligated to begin a resuscitation attempt on all patients who suffer a cardiac arrest unless a 'do not attempt resuscitation' (DNAR) status has been agreed. Although a nurse could cite moral grounds for refusing to resuscitate a patient without a DNAR order this could be to earn institutional, legal and professional censure and might lead to professional sanction including the possibility of dismissal and the loss of a licence to practice. Given that a nurse is expected to know these things and while it might seem to be a moral act to refuse to take an active part in an inappropriate resuscitation attempt, under normal circumstances the more moral act would be to pre-empt inappropriate resuscitation attempts by arguing for a DNAR order. Task or response training then may well be appropriate for some aspects of the role of a nurse but such training is not without moral significance.

Training then has moral implications but it is not moral training as such. Moral training implies being trained to act in particular ways that others believe to be morally correct and in relation to the ends or goals of those same others. A distinction between training and education is made here and hinges on the idea of human moral agency. It is possible to train a dog to perform certain tricks or to train a parrot to say certain words but in so acting (so far as we know) neither the dog nor the parrot are engaging with moral agency. So we might train our paratrooper and our nurse to do certain things but even in so doing we accept that neither will do these things without retaining their capacity for moral agency.

Towards an understanding of moral education for nurses

So we can say that moral education is different from moral training because in moral education we aim to assist individuals to recognise and develop their moral agency. If the purpose of nursing education is to enable nurses to engage in nursing as a practice then, because this involves the cultivation of particular virtues, education for nursing is a form of moral education. Thinking of nurse education as a form of moral education serves to remind us of the interconnectedness of ideas and actions, of reason and emotion, and of character and behaviour. It serves, in MacIntyre's terms, to reduce the fragmentation of modernity. Thus while the education of nurses involves some training (as noted above) as well as the learning of propositional and practical knowledge this must all take place within a recognition of the aims and scope of nursing practice. And if the practice of nursing is, as I have claimed, primarily concerned with human betterment then it matters a great deal not only what nurses do but also the manner in which they go about doing it. In other words, the safe and competent completion of tasks alone is insufficient to define good nursing. Rather good nursing requires the safe and competent completion of tasks undertaken with an explicit regard for the well-being of patients. That is, good nursing requires a good will (in the strong sense) and the cultivation of the virtues.

Teaching for good will and the virtues

If the above is true then those involved in the teaching of nurses (let us call them 'nurse teachers' for the time being) will need to work out how it might be best to go about teaching for good will (in the strong sense) and the virtues. It would be a mistake to imagine there might be a simple, ready-made pedagogy available for nurse teachers merely to adopt as a teaching method in order to achieve this aim. For this would be to assume teaching is no more than the application of method whereas, as stated in the opening chapter of this book, teaching, like nursing, is a complex professional and moral practice, a practice moreover that can be described in MacIntyrean terms. One implication of this is that if we are serious about teaching nurses to engage with nursing as a practice then nurse teachers can go some way towards this aim by engaging in a practice (or practices) themselves. In so doing nurse teachers can begin to illustrate what it is to pursue the goods internal to a practice. That is to say that if nurse teachers are engaged in teaching as a practice then it becomes possible for students to imagine how engaging with a practice, rather than merely undertaking a set of tasks, might bring with it goods other than external goods. I will return to this later in this chapter, for now it is necessary to outline the sorts of questions raised by the idea that the purpose of teaching for nursing is teaching for good will and for the virtue.

Teaching for good will

Teaching that aims for the development of good will (in the strong sense) in students of nursing requires that nurse teachers have a clear idea of what good will entails. As indicated earlier in this chapter and also in Chapter 4, good will requires more than mere well-meaning intention for it is commonplace that well-meaning intentions can very easily lead to harm. If we assume that well-meaning intention is akin to everyday understandings of altruism, and given that there is at least anecdotal evidence to suggest that those who become students of nursing generally do so because they want to help others, then we might say that the students in front of us are students of the 'right sort' and will want to put their well-meaning intentions to good use. Just as Aristotle suggests that those young men who already have some understanding of the importance of being noble and just will gain most from his lectures on ethics (Burnyeat 1984) so we might say that those students who already have some nascent conception of nursing as a practice (or at least as an activity with some worthwhile internal goods) will be most receptive to ideas about nursing as a professional ideal requiring certain sorts of dispositions. If this is true then the selection of students for nursing becomes a matter of considerable consequence for the practice of nursing will be best served by recruiting those with appropriate altruistic emotions and dispositions. But as a raw emotion, there is nothing about altruism per se that gives us grounds for confidence that it alone can guide professional practice. In this sense altruism shares the issue highlighted in Chapter 1 in relation to virtue. That is, that life in our (often) comfortable liberal democracies does not provide challenges to our altruistic emotions sufficient to develop these emotions in ways that can help us to act morally when faced with extra-ordinary challenges. Thus something that should be of serious concern to nurse teachers is the question of how we might go about enabling students to turn their altruistic intentions into good will. The practitioner with good will in the strong sense will recognise the limitations of mere well-meant intentions; will recognise that to turn such intentions into good will requires that a genuine regard for the welfare of others must be augmented by a well-informed approach to their practice.

Teaching for the virtues

Dunne (1999) reminds us that in response to Socrates' question about whether virtue can be taught, Aristotle tells us that while teaching is appropriate for the development of intellectual virtues, the cultivation of moral virtue lies in habituation. In seeking guidance from Aristotle about how we might go about encouraging the development of moral virtue in others by the use of habituation, Dunne notes Aristotle's own ambiguity in describing *phronesis* as an intellectual virtue in the *Nicomachean Ethics* while leaving it out of discussions of the intellectual virtues elsewhere. The eccentricity (as Dunne calls it) of *phronesis* is writ large if we accept Aristotle's categorisation of it in the *Nicomachean Ethics* as an intellectual virtue and thus, in Aristotle's own scheme, teachable as any other intellectual virtue. Dunne notes that it cannot be just one intellectual virtue among others because it is of central importance in Aristotle's account. *Phronesis* (practical wisdom) is the exercise of judgement enabling us to know what to do to whom, in what measure in what way and at what time. This is to say that the expression of moral virtue requires *phronesis*. In addition, as Dunne puts it 'ethical virtue is itself required for *phronesis*. If a clever person is not good, neither will he be a *phronimos* (practically wise person)' (Dunne 1999, p.50; original emphasis).

As Dunne further notes, for Aristotle there is nothing to be gained from the pursuit of moral knowledge in the absence of seeking to become moral. For Aristotle the point of learning more about, for example, justice lies in a genuine desire to become just and to act justly. And being just requires not only being disposed to be just but also learning to recognise what justice requires in different situations. The person who knows what the virtues require in different situations is the *phronimos*. Yet the teaching conundrum remains, for in our time the value placed on theoretical knowledge (the universals in Aristotelian terms) drives the educational enterprise. By and large, the measurement of knowledge throughout our educational system is geared to and rewards the demonstration of theoretical knowledge. It is this separation to which MacIntyre so objects and he does so for Aristotelian reasons. In part this separation is inevitable given our seeming inability to assess practical knowledge in the kinds of systematic ways that the current climate of audit culture demands. Even in practice-based work (such as nursing) the difficulties of measuring practical knowledge remain unresolved. And if most nursing students (like most other students) are assessment driven then this separation between theory and practice (between, in Aristotelian terms, universals and particulars) is likely to increase rather than decrease.

By definition then any educational process that aims to encourage the development of virtue (including most importantly *phronesis*) must also aim to work towards instilling in the student an understanding of the intimate relationship between the universals and the particulars in a practice-based discipline such as nursing. While knowledge of the universals (propositional knowledge) is necessary for safe and competence practice, propositional knowledge on its own will not make for good practice in relation to a particular patient in a particular situation at a particular time. Similarly, effective practical technique or mere task competence without some sort of underpinning propositional knowledge is an impoverished and undesirable basis for nursing practice. This is something Florence Nightingale understood as witnessed by her recognition that nurses should not merely act from unthinking obedience despite her general requirement that nurses obey doctors' orders (Nightingale 1952). Although she insisted on *training* for probationers (student nurses would be the nearest modern equivalent), Nightingale was very clear that nurses needed to develop a great deal of practical wisdom if they were to make a positive difference for the patients in their care. In part, her use of the word training reflects both the social and language conventions of the day and should not lead us to suppose that she necessarily meant by it what we would understand by it today. Nevertheless, this recognition of the necessity to understand the close relationship between what we now tend to classify as propositional and practical knowledge in practice-based occupations such as nursing is an essential part of engaging with nursing as a practice. Indeed, one feature of understanding nursing as a practice is that it provides a logical way of understanding knowledge in a less polarised fashion. As well as enabling us to situate the values inherent in theoretical knowledge within a framework of the traditions of a practice, a practice allows us to overcome the overly simplistic idea that practical nursing knowledge is merely the application of scientific propositional knowledge in practical situations. As such, nursing (like any other practice) provides a way in which the world of the universals (the academy) and the world of the particulars (everyday nursing practice) can move closer together. This need not be in any physical sense although that is not precluded; rather it is a closeness that permeates the work of both. And it is not merely that each should recognise the contribution of the other; rather it is the recognition that each is engaged in only one part of a much larger enterprise.

Teaching for intellectual virtue

In his 1999 paper Dunne is self-consciously attempting to fathom how we might, as teachers, use Aristotelian habituation to encourage others to cultivate moral virtue. But the same scrutiny of teaching for intellectual virtue might reveal that we have much work to do to understand how *any* virtue (be it intellectual or moral) may be taught. While Aristotle talks of the time and experience necessary for the teaching of intellectual virtue and in contrast the use of habituation in the pursuit of moral virtue, it is far from obvious that habituation is not involved in the cultivation of both precisely because it is far from clear that the separation of intellectual and moral virtues is established. Indeed, Steutel and Spiecker (2005) suggest that there might be a stronger prima facie case for thinking that habituation is better suited to enabling the cultivation of intellectual virtue (in the form of *habits of the mind*) than it is in cultivation of what they term sentimental dispositions.

In many ways it is helpful to maintain a distinction between the intellectual and moral domains but we might be well advised to resist the temptation to imagine this categorisation provides us with full understanding of virtue. It may well be the case that, as with the infant who confuses cats with dogs, the criteria we use in the categorisation process are insufficiently discriminating. It may serve us well as part of coming to understand phenomena but as we know from our educational experiences, learning is largely iterative and the more deeply immersed we become in a subject the more we begin to recognise the inherent contradictions within the subject and the more we understand the limitations of our knowledge. And so it may be with virtue. Dunne's portrayal of *phronesis* as eccentric may be true insofar as it is centrally important but it is not without possibility that we might make a similar case for, for example, open-mindedness. Indeed we might go so far as to suggest that at least some of the other virtues are eccentric on the grounds that they may not be so easily identifiable as solely virtues of the intellect or the character (again, open-mindedness is a candidate to illustrate this point).

Unsurprisingly, in the same way that teaching that aims for the development of good will requires teachers to have a clear idea of what good will entails, teaching that aims for the development of virtue in students of nursing requires that nurse teachers aim to develop an understanding of the nature of virtue. And given that virtue remains a contested notion we must allow that this is no easy task. It is, however, a task that we might find easier when we aim to engage with teaching as a practice in the MacIntyrean sense.

Teaching for the moral practice of nursing

It will be noticed that the headings of the last few sections indicate teaching *for* rather than the teaching *of*. This deliberate choice of words reflects the view that teaching as a practice has more to do with helping others to learn than with the mere transmission of information from teacher to student. It will also be noticed here that the focus of the discussion has moved from teaching to learning. Again this is deliberate for it is a well-worn truism that however skilful a teacher might be (given that we are talking about education rather than training or indoctrination) any learning that takes place is as much, if not more of, a function of the student's willingness to learn as it is of the ability of the teacher to teach. If this is right then the practice of teaching for nursing must aim in the first instance to enable students to learn what learning to be a nurse requires of them. From this perspective we need no longer be preoccupied with whether or not virtue can be taught and can turn our attention to that part of Socrates' question about the acquisition of virtue which is perhaps more germane, that is, whether virtue can be learned.

As I have noted elsewhere (Sellman 2009) this manoeuvre is one used by Gilbert Ryle (1972) although for Ryle it is born from a recognition of the similarities between learning language and learning about virtue. According to Ryle because we learn both language and virtue (or vice) as we grow then it must be true that both language and virtue can be taught, although it is not taught in the way we think of formal teaching as represented in schools and colleges. If Ryle is right about this then teaching aimed at enabling others to become moral takes place at the informal level 'as we seek first to imitate and then later to emulate those around us whom we admire' (Sellman 2009, p.89). On this account our teachers are not (or at least not solely) our professors rather our teachers are all around us and we learn from them in subtle, unplanned, and unexpected ways – although we can and do take guidance either deliberately or by something not dissimilar to a form of osmosis from those who surround us as we go about our daily lives.

Identifying the nurse teachers

Up to this point I have been using the term 'nurse teacher' rather indiscriminately and it is now time to review this potentially misleading nomenclature. There are many who are involved in teaching nurses and while it is true that many of those formally employed (predominantly within institutions of higher education) to teach nurses are themselves nurses there are others who are not. It may be that any one or more of the discrete disciplines of anatomy and physiology, psychology, sociology, ethics, law and so on might be taught not by nurses but by academics from those disciplines. It is possible that, for example, the person teaching sociology to nurses might be a sociologist with an interest in teaching nurses, a sociologist with a sociological interest in nursing, a nurse with an interest (and, perhaps, an appropriate qualification) in sociology, or both a nurse and a sociologist. In addition, while many who teach nurses in the academy are themselves nurses many of them will not teach nursing as such. This is partly related to the contested nature of nursing knowledge and partly to do with the fact that many nurse teachers who are nurses have become specialist teachers of, for example, anatomy and physiology, research, ethics and so on insofar as these subjects relate to nursing. Thus even in the academy those who teach nurses will not necessarily be nurses nor will they necessarily be teaching nursing as such, hence the misleading nature of the term nurse teacher. A nurse teacher might be a nurse and a teacher (although not necessarily teach nursing), might be a teacher who happens to teach a subject of relevance to nurses, or might be a nurse who teaches nursing. Different arrangements occur in different institutions across the globe, often for no other reason than historical accident or the local availability of academics from other disciplines.

But, as has already been observed, nursing is a practice-based discipline and arguably the nurse teachers with the most influence on students of nursing are the practitioners themselves. Indeed, it is a requirement made explicit in many nursing codes that registered practitioners have an obligation to facilitate the learning of those who seek to become future registered nurses, although the extent to which this injunction has settled into the general consciousness of the working population of nurses themselves remains to be seen. For it is the case that the traditional division between 'theory' and 'practice' remains and provides one of the recognised stressors of pre-registration nursing students as they try to negotiate appropriate 'student' type behaviour in each of these two very different learning environments as they move between the academy and practice placements.

It seems, then, that there are three broad categories of nurse teachers, each with a slightly different primary function. The first group can be distinguished as those whose primary function lies in the delivery of nursing care to patients, and although these practitioners of nursing have a professional obligation to enable students to learn, few will understand this as a primary or even a priority task in the face of the competing demands of proving safe and effective care. The second group of nurse teachers are usually registered nurses employed specifically in educational roles within clinically facing organisations (hospitals and other health care facilities and so on) to operationalise or develop educational policies within those institutions. Such roles develop in different ways in different practice areas and some have specific responsibility for the educational and training needs of nurses and student nurses, others have much wider institutional roles. The third group of nurse teachers are those who are employed in institutions of higher education as teachers of nursing or other specific subjects relevant to the education of nurses.

In the UK the terms *mentor, practice educator,* and *lecturer* have been identified as appropriate for registered nurses who fall within the first, second and third of these groups of nurse teachers respectively (English National Board for Nursing, Midwifery and Health Visiting and Department of Health 2001) and henceforth I shall use these terms to differentiate between the three groups. I will continue to use nurse teacher as an umbrella term to indicate those included in all three groups. Thus:

> If Ryle is correct to say that our teachers of morality are those whom we admire and attempt to emulate, then it becomes incumbent on those who mentor nursing students to strive to be practitioners of the sort we would want those learning the practice to become. Hence…it may not be necessary for practitioners to try to teach *phronesis* at all; rather, the mentors need to (merely) exemplify what the role encompasses. (Sellman 2009, p.89)

In moral terms this means being honest, just, courageous, trustworthy and open-minded so that it offers the student a glimpse of what moral practice requires. Those who are sufficiently moved to wish to convert their raw altruistic emotions and their well-meaning intentions into informed good will in order to best meet the moral requirements of nursing will wish to emulate those traits of character they see as admirable both for their own sake and for their contribution to the flourishing of *more-than-ordinarily* vulnerable persons. This may also work in reverse insofar as our well-meaning student may witness unedifying actions that hinder the flourishing of *more-than-ordinarily* vulnerable persons and by the same token may work towards ensuring they do not emulate those vices.

Steutel and Spiecker claim that the tutor who takes on the role of a mentor is the essential ingredient of an Aristotelian habituation in the inculcation of moral virtue. They note that habituation may be an entirely appropriate way of developing habits but that the case for habituation leading to the cultivation of affective dispositions is much harder to make. They say:

> the relationship between consistently doing the proper things and the establishment of corresponding habits is quite easy to grasp, whereas a relationship between such a way of learning and acquiring sentimental dispositions is difficult to fathom. Doing virtuous things on a regular basis is likely to result in virtuous habits, but how could such a practice also result in dispositions to be affected in virtuous ways? (Steutel and Spiecker 2005, p.540)

Of course, this raises an essential difference between the aims of moral education generally in which the teacher is attempting to inculcate dispositions in those who may not be disposed to value those dispositions, and the aims of moral education for nursing (at least as I am framing it here) where the teacher is attempting to encourage students to develop enduring traits of character (at least in professional life) in those who are assumed to have the appropriate, if raw, altruistic emotions. Nevertheless, their claim that habituation in the attempt to inculcate moral virtue can only be successful with the supervision of a virtuous tutor is readily translatable to nursing education. And the fact that the professional body for nursing in the UK has chosen as the preferred term mentor, to denote the practising nurse whose primary role is in direct patient care, suggests just this view of the nurse as a guide for the learner; as someone whose nursing practice is admirable (in the sense of being admired); and as a practitioner the student might seek to emulate in order to become themselves an admirable nurse. This returns us to the *professional phronimos*.

The *professional phronimos* as nurse teacher

Inherent in the above discussion is the idea that those nurse teachers who engage with their work as a practice exemplify what it is to be a *professional phronimos*. The mentor will be engaged with nursing as a practice (which essentially includes the facilitation of student learning), the practice educator and the lecturer will be engaged with teaching as a practice. In both cases those who engage with their professional work as a practice will exemplify those traits of character, those dispositions, those virtues that are constitutive of their work as a practice. This *professional phronimos* (the professionally practically wise person) is one who genuinely cares about the standards that, in MacIntyre's terms, are constitutive of the practice with which they are engaged. They aim for excellence in the practice and have adopted or developed methods to help them pursue the excellences of the practice. They may have learned to become reflexive about their practice, that is, they may have habituated themselves to think about their practice in terms of how far their actions have enabled rather than hindered the flourishing of *more-than-ordinarily* vulnerable persons. The particular tools they have used to develop mastery of their practice matter less than the effective use of those tools and if they are able to articulate in words, actions and sentiments how they continue to learn to master their practice in ways that the student can understand then the student has an opportunity of learning what engaging with the practice requires of them. They will see the practitioner not only acting in ways that aim for the benefit of patients but also see how the practitioner ensures their altruistic emotions work for the benefit rather than to the detriment of the patient. They will see that the admirable practitioner is (or strives to be) honest, just, courageous, trustworthy and open-minded and will see how these enduring characteristics contribute in essential ways to engagement in a practice. In addition, the mentor can demonstrate how she or he uses tools such as reflection in everyday practice as a way of enhancing that practice and in so doing can help the learner to avoid the trap of mistaking the use of such a tool as an end in itself.

For lecturers who are engaged in the practice of teaching as a way of enabling learners to learn to become engaged in the practice of nursing there are pedagogic and curriculum implications. The lecturer who exemplifies the practice of teaching will similarly illustrate to students something about how being engaged with a practice has internal goods that are worth striving for. In addition, the lecturer will have genuine concerns about how far pedagogic and curriculum arrangements enable rather than hinder the development of learners towards the ideal of the *professional phronimos*. In this sense, teachers as facilitators of learning (rather than as transmitters of information) will seek to develop pedagogies that are student-centred, that encourage deep rather than surface learning, and that enable learners to develop as learners. This is particularly important in a practice-based occupation such as nursing because remaining a safe and competent practitioner requires skills of lifelong learning together with an openness to challenges to current practice and a willingness to adopt changes in practice in the light of compelling evidence. Teaching methods that may encourage these things will include, but are not limited to, approaches such as peer and self-appraisal and assessment, work-based learning, problem-based learning (sometimes referred to as enquiry or context based learning), seminars and so on. This is to say that it includes any teaching method that moves away from an over-reliance on didactic lectures as the primary method of instruction (although we should not forget that there is, of course, a place for lectures within an overall pedagogy that encourages active student learning). What these teaching approaches have in common is the ideological canon that inclines learners to participate as active learners, to participate in making judgements, and towards less reliance on the teacher as an expert. The lecturer may be an expert in their subject area as a subject area but for a practice-based occupation where what might be a right action is in some sense inevitably contextual, the best the lecturer can offer might be a way of ensuring that things the practitioner ought to take into consideration when making a decision are not neglected. And further, if it is true as I have intimated in this book that students do tend to be assessment driven, lecturers should aim to ensure that the assessments assess that which we wish the student to demonstrate and that this includes their capacity to make reasoned moral judgements in practice situations. Moreover, the assessments ought to be such that students are encouraged to learn in ways that will help them to continue to learn once they are qualified practitioners.

Competences

Where there is a tendency among those working in nursing education to concentrate on the easily measurable, that this often takes the form of task competences. It may seem odd that nursing, as a practice-based profession has felt the need to emphasise task competence (in the narrow sense) in professional education for it might be thought that anyone who wants to become a nurse would recognise immediately the necessity for safe and competent practice. Yet the idea of competence in task in nursing is moot. The problem is related to a general perception (at least in some quarters) that nursing is a simple occupation that anyone can do. Anecdotal evidence suggests that there is a widely held belief among nurses, students of nursing, health care assistants (and, unsurprisingly perhaps, many students are drawn from the ranks of health care assistants) and others that while nursing is hard physical work there is little else involved; an often voiced opinion that theory is largely irrelevant for practice; and a general view that even the 'simple' physical tasks of nursing require little education or training. There seems to be an almost institutionalised anti-intellectualism amongst some practitioners as expressed in these views and evidenced (perhaps) by the repeatedly recorded barriers to implementing changes in practice even where such changes have overwhelming support from research evidence (see, for example, Hek *et al.* 2002) and the resistance to manual handling as discussed in Chapter 5 provides one telling example.

This emphasis on the teaching and measurement of task competence is, of course, an essential aspect of an education that aims to prepare students to become safe practitioners and it reflects the current prominence of the evidence-based practice movement. But if we mistake this approach for a full account of nursing education then we neglect the crucial human experience of health and illness. If the purpose of nursing is, as I have claimed, to enable the flourishing of *more-than-ordinarily* vulnerable persons then a concentration on task competence understates the importance of human frailty. If I am right about this then the practice of nurse education must seek to encompass the cultivation of the virtues of nursing.

I have already suggested that in teaching for virtue nurse teachers can illustrate virtue in action in their own everyday practice and this can alert students to possibilities about the rewarding nature of the internal goods of a practice. Thus far the discussion has remained at an abstract level. In the final section of this chapter I shall offer a brief discussion about some of the particulars of this aretiac virtue ethics approach to the moral education of nurses.

Teaching for trustworthiness and open-mindedness

We have seen that if the nurse teacher is engaged in teaching *as a practice* then they will approximate what I have termed the *professional phronimos* and what Steutel and Spiecker call the virtuous tutor. In their conception of Aristotelian habituation it is the virtuous tutor who can help the learner to learn what it is that virtue requires of them and this is important because merely learning to habitually *act as if* one were honest, just or courageous only serves the limited purpose of moral training. And as we have seen moral training does not take sufficient account of human moral agency. If it were possible to train a student to *always* tell the truth then we will have failed that student by repressing her or his moral agency. For she or he will have not been given the opportunity to exercise judgement and discretion. Even on a Kantian account, mere training of moral habits denies moral agency because without a rational understanding of the 'rule' of truth telling, the mere act of rule following has no moral force. Whereas it is part of the conception of the *professional phronimos* that she or he has the wisdom to recognise what the exercise of a virtue requires in a particular situation. The virtuous tutor then illustrates by what she or he does in everyday practice the exercise of the virtues necessary for that practice. In this way the *professional phronimos* will not only seek to enable the student to learn the 'facts' of trustworthiness but also what trustworthiness requires; will not only teach the student what open-mindedness is but also how to go about being open-minded. This can take various forms but one essential aspect involves teaching the student that there are judgements to be made in the exercise of both trustworthiness and open-mindedness and the way that the virtuous tutor goes about being trustworthy and open-minded in different situations is instructive.

Learning to be trustworthy

Being trustworthy will be instructive in the first instance in the relationship between the nurse teacher and the student. As Nancy Potter (2002) points out one thing that being trustworthy requires of us is that we respond in trustworthy ways to betrayals of trust; that we make sincere attempts to recover trust when trust relationships have broken down. We can betray a trust in many ways and in some cases we may not even be aware of the breach. We may break a trust inadvertently when, for example, we are striving to learn to be trustworthy; we may break a trust deliberately in professional life as we face situations in which a breach of trust is justified or inevitable; or we may breach a trust without realising that the other party has placed their trust in us. Arguably, the nature of professional working life is such that unasked for or unacknowledged trust may accompany unrealistic or unreasonable expectations of patients about what is and what is not within the scope of a professional's role to accomplish. Thorne and Robinson illustrate this in their study of patients with chronic illness who:

> entered into health care relationships with an almost absolute trust in the professionals who would provide care. This initial trust was based on the naïve assumption that answers to their health care problems would be forthcoming and that the health care professional would be singularly dedicated to providing them with those answers. (Thorne and Robinson 1988, p.783)

What these patients found was that, in time and with an emergent understanding of the health care system, their expectations of the health care professionals became more realistic in terms of what the professionals could or could not offer, or, to put this another way, became more realistic in terms of how far they could trust the health care professional to look after their best interests. The situation is likely to be similar in other professional relationships such as those between a learner and a teacher.

In the same way that a nurse who finds she or he must betray the trust of a patient,[21] the nurse teacher who finds she or he has betrayed students' trust must make genuine attempts at reparation. Admitting that one has broken a trust entails being honest, just and courageous. It takes honesty to recognise the part one played in a breach of trust, it takes an understanding of what justice requires to recognise that being untrustworthy (even in a single instance) is to be unfair, and it takes courage to admit to one's role in a betrayal of trust. And because genuine attempts at a repair of broken trust require the admission of fault, actions that aim at reparation illustrate the expression of those three virtues. And the receptive learner, that is, the student or registered nurse who aims to become trustworthy, can learn from the nurse teacher not only how difficult it is to be trustworthy but also how the virtuous person might go about recovering a lost trust in a virtuous way. Similarly, the virtuous mentor will exemplify trustworthiness in the practice of nursing. As illustrated in Chapter 4, dilemmas of trustworthiness are more likely in practice situations precisely because the practitioner must answer to a number of different individuals or groups. The way in which the *professional phronimos* negotiates the difficulties of being trustworthy in everyday practice settings will illustrate to the willing learner the relative importance the virtuous mentor places on each competing demand of trustworthiness. In short, the virtuous mentor illustrates to the student that learning to become trustworthy requires learning to be honest, just and courageous.

Learning to be open-minded

I have outlined elsewhere some suggestions for how learning to be open-minded might proceed as part of a discussion on teaching for *professional phronesis* (Sellman 2009), here I will summarise and add to some of those suggestions. First though some background information to set the scene.

As McLaughlin (2003b) points out, it would be odd to imagine that teachers set out deliberately to encourage students to become closed-minded or credulous rather than open-minded. And yet, as I have argued, closed-minded and credulous nurses are known to exist, and presumably are to be found among the ranks of those I have identified as nurse teachers. As outlined in Chapter 5, being open-minded is not to be equated with having no firm beliefs and thus learning to be open-minded requires learning to hold beliefs in an open-minded way. It would seem axiomatic that if the nurse teacher claims to be open-minded but in some way fails to be open-minded then the student will perceive hypocrisy in operation, even if it is the case that the teacher is self-deluded in thinking her or himself open-minded. From this it would seem apparent that the open-minded teacher or nurse is one who both demonstrates open-mindedness in action and encourages the learner to be similarly open-minded. The ideal of open-mindedness for practice appears to be an educational imperative in any occupation (such as nursing) that is serious in its pursuit of evidence-based practice. Open-mindedness is essential for evidence-based practice precisely because basing practice on evidence not only presupposes that practitioners are sufficiently open-minded to engage with new evidence which might refute rather than support existing practice but also that practitioners are willing to change practice on the basis of compelling evidence. This is no small matter for it requires the practitioner to acknowledge that their own practice may turn out to be incorrect, which in turn requires an honest appraisal of current practice in the light of an honest appraisal of new evidence.

In some ways teaching for open-mindedness is easier than teaching for trustworthiness (at least for the nurse teacher who is generally disposed to be open-minded) as the teacher can embody what it is to be open-minded: in addition the teacher can set tasks that lead learners towards being open-minded. In the classroom such tasks might include, for example, requiring learners to adopt positions contrary to their own strongly held beliefs in order to engage in debate about fundamental questions relating to nursing. Set up as formal debates with proposers and opposers arguing from a rational perspective for and against extreme positions, this can encourage learners to engage more deeply than they otherwise would with the logic of opposing positions on a range of topical and perhaps, but not necessarily, controversial issues of relevance to practice. Of course, such debates need not be related to nursing if the aim is merely to develop particular intellectual habits of mind (those habits that encourage rather than discourage open-mindedness) but there is a case to be made for sustaining a relevance in order to direct those habits of mind towards the general aim of nursing education: that is, to enable as far is possible the flourishing of *more-than-ordinarily* vulnerable persons.

Similarly, and even in formal learning and teaching situations, the application of critical habits of mind by the teacher in relation to whatever subject is under discussion allows the learner to see for themselves what aiming for open-mindedness looks like – and those learners who are convinced of the desirability of open-mindedness can seek to emulate those features of open-mindedness they see in the way their teacher approaches the subject. And if the teacher is explicit about what sorts of questions she or he asks of whatever topic is under consideration, and why those and not other questions, then the learner can begin to approach situations as well as theoretical concepts with a similar inquisitiveness. In this sense at least, the habituation that

Aristotle suggests as the way to develop virtue seems to offer a route for learners in learning to become open-minded.

Thus, education for *professional phronesis* in nursing is a form of moral education and requires that nurse teachers take seriously their obligations in this respect. The nature of this moral education is to be distinguished from moral training which, while superficially attractive, cannot function to develop *phronesis* precisely because it neglects to account for moral agency. And moral agency is necessary if nurses are to be, or are to become, autonomous and accountable practitioners. This idea of the nurse as an autonomous and accountable practitioner is generally accepted as appropriate and is clearly articulated in nursing codes, although what this means for the education of nurses is largely neglected. As a consequence, while the teaching of ethics has become an accepted requirement of nurse education, the issue of the moral education of nurses is insufficiently emphasised. Yet without a recognition of the moral nature of nurse education, those enduring character dispositions that we anticipate will be exhibited by nurses will not be perceived as part of the province of nurse teachers and will thus remain neglected by those with the potential to influence (in systematic ways and for the benefit of *more-than-ordinarily* vulnerable persons) successive generations of nurses.

Conclusion

In this book I have begun an exploration of some of the virtues necessary for nursing practice. I have argued that there is good reason for nurses to develop inter alia the virtues of honesty, justice, courage, trustworthiness, open-mindedness and, perhaps most importantly, what I have termed *professional phronesis* tailored and appropriate to the practice of nursing. As a result it is incumbent on nurse teachers to provide students with both the opportunities to cultivate these virtues and the environments that permit the expression of these virtues. Nursing (and nurse education/teaching) conceived as a practice in the technical sense in which MacIntyre employs that term helps to provide the kinds of environment in which these educational goals can be pursued in ways that avoid some of the tensions between means and ends. Further, the notion of nursing as a practice is especially helpful in the pursuit of the moral aims of nursing education because of the focus on internal rather than external goods.

I have rehearsed the idea that patients are *more-than-ordinarily* vulnerable precisely because they are patients and that nursing conceived as a practice is intimately involved with enabling human flourishing. I have offered an exploration of the place of trustworthiness and open-mindedness as professional virtues specific to the practice of nursing and discussed how the development of these dispositions in nurses can contribute to the aim of enabling the flourishing of *more-than-ordinarily* vulnerable persons. I have suggested that while altruism may be a desirable quality in those who seek to become nurses, it is generally a raw altruistic emotion that can only function in beneficial ways if cultivated within a framework of virtue and reason. To know what to do, when, in what way and for what reason requires practical wisdom and not merely technical or intellectual capacities. Thus the development of the practically wise nurse (the *professional phronimos*) is a proper aim of nursing education and an education that seeks to develop the *professional phronimos* is a moral education. Hence, the idea of a moral education for nursing is of considerable importance and it is an idea that all nurse teachers must take seriously if students are to be enabled to develop the sorts of characteristics that are expected of nurses. It is within this framework that the teaching of nursing takes place and within which subject specialist teachers (including teachers of ethics) can contribute towards the goal of the *professional phronimos*.

I have explored elsewhere (Sellman 2007) some of the limitations and potential tensions regarding the possibilities of evaluating the good character of students and registrants. Here I merely observe that there are issues raised by the requirement of many nursing regulatory bodies (including the Nursing and Midwifery Council) that, as well as passing an officially approved programme of education leading to nurse registration, those who apply to join a register of nurses should be of good character. In the UK this declaration must be signed by a registered nurse who holds an appropriately responsible position within the institution where the course of study has been undertaken by the applicant. The declaration confirms that: '**to the best of my knowledge**...[I] believe the above named student's health and character are sufficiently good to enable safe and effective practice and that there is an intention to comply with the *Code*...' (NMC undated; original emphasis). This declaration of good character is significant for without it the aspiring registrant is unable to gain a license to practice. Yet it is not clear that those with responsibility for programmes of nurse education have this aim in mind when developing the nursing curriculum. It seems that signing the declaration of good character is not something that nurse educators worry about despite the flimsy guidance offered by nursing's regulatory bodies in regard to what is to be taken into account when making such an assessment.

The work of this book is offered as a contribution to the understanding of what is required if a nurse is to be of good character. We might say that a nurse of good character can be relied upon to act *characteristically* in ways that enhance the flourishing of patients. That is to say that a nurse of good character is one who is disposed towards compassion, caring, honesty, a sense of fairness and so on, in short, has the sorts of dispositions that are considered necessary for good nursing. And further, that these dispositions are of an enduring nature and can be cultivated as virtues appropriate for the practice of nursing. So the nurse of good character has, or at least strives towards, the virtues of justice, courage and honesty, as well as the professional virtues of trustworthiness, open-mindedness and *professional phronesis*.

The declaration of good health and good character required in the UK by the NMC also assumes that nurse teachers are able and qualified to make judgements about how far a student intends, once registered, to comply with the NMC Code (NMC 2008b). This idea is consistent with the thrust of the injunctions of regulatory bodies in general and of the NMC in particular. There is a sense, however, in which it is expected that a nurse freely chooses to comply with their code and in so doing expresses moral agency. Without this, complying with the code takes the form of a moral training that seems somewhat inconsistent with the requirement that nurses should be autonomous and accountable ethical practitioners. Yet the authoritarian functions of nursing's regulatory bodies requires that they measure the behaviour of individual nurses against a nursing code whether or not those nurses have accepted the tenets of their code. This gives rise to a paradox seemingly lost on those who hold regulatory authority over nurses. For if it is the case that nurses are expected to adopt the values of their code then such acceptance needs to occur as a result of free choice (for without this it lacks moral force); yet the sanctions that regulatory bodies can apply mitigate against the virtues outlined in this book precisely because without those virtues there is no reason (apart from the fear of losing one's licence to practice) for nurses to adhere to the tenets of their code. Hence, the requirement for an ethical practitioner is a requirement for the moral education of nurses and not merely for compliance with a set of loosely stated principles of practice. O'Hear puts this succinctly after noting that moral education is about enabling freely chosen internalisation and recognising that this leads to the authoritarian problem of 'how a moral educator can avoid being an authoritarian indoctrinator, trying to enforce a morality on an agent who should ideally be freely and rationally deciding for himself' (O'Hear 1998, p.15). Thus those involved in the education of nurses cannot ignore the fact that their own practice (be it nursing or teaching practice) has an impact, for good or ill, on the moral development of nursing students. For moral education is not the province of specialist teachers of morality but is part of the fabric of the environment in which learning to become a nurse takes place. Only some of this learning to become a nurse will occur as part of the formal educational curriculum where students pursue achievement of pre-set and detailed learning outcomes. It is the morality of the academy and of health care *as institutions* together with the morality of individual practitioners as much as, or perhaps even instead of, the teachings of nurse teachers (be they mentors, practice educators or lecturers) that shapes student nurses' understanding of the morality of nursing practice. This means that students' internalisation of their code is most likely where this does not lead to dissonance between the virtue requirements and the values inherent in the code on the one hand and, on the other, those values and virtues (or vices) they see actualised by the nurses and nurse teachers they work with in everyday practice. Similarly, nurses and nurse teachers will be more likely to have internalised the tenets of the code where institutional arrangements encourage rather than discourage the expression of those tenets. Thus, the general morality of the institutions of health care provision and of health care education have an important part to play in the moral education of nurses. Both MacIntyre (1985) and Potter (2002) warn of the potential for institutional arrangements to undermine ethical practice and those nurse teachers who emphasise managerial ideals at the expense of professional ideals of service (those, in MacIntyre's terms, who pursue the goods of effectiveness at the cost of the goods of excellence) will not only distort the traditions of nursing as a practice but will also add to the dissonance students experience between the code and practice.

As intimated in Chapter 1, the idea of internalisation suggests that as well as a requirement for knowledge of their nursing code, education for nursing should aim to inculcate in students the values inherent in that code in order that they characteristically behave in particular ways; particular ways, that is, that can reasonably be assumed to be part of what the regulatory body understands as being of good character. But if this is to be more than mere indoctrination then students need to be convinced that being of good character is a necessary aspect of ensuring their altruistic emotions are developed for the benefit rather than to the detriment of patients. This is to say, that students need to be convinced that a good nurse is one who has cultivated those virtues identified as necessary for the practice of nursing.

There is a great deal of further work to be done about the meaning of good character as well as in relation to the how and when of its measurement in students and practitioners of nursing. Becoming an ethical practitioner is indeed a noble aim but this aim does not yet seem to be translated in explicit ways into the curriculum; further it is a noble idea about which nurses themselves appear to experience some ambiguity. Certainly what nursing's regulatory bodies understand by the moral requirements of being of good character is insufficiently spelled out. It is my sincere hope that this book makes a positive contribution to the debate about what we understand as being of good character, as well as a further positive contribution to our understanding of what an education that explicitly aims to produce such nurses would involve.

Endnotes

1   There are isolated examples of ethics teaching to nurses before this: for example, Alistair Campbell (a theologian) was delivering ethics lectures to nurses in Scotland in the 1970s. However, the point here is that with the introduction of Project 2000 it was nurse teachers who found themselves having to deliver the ethics component of the nursing curriculum. One course aimed specifically at nurse teachers teaching ethics without any formal qualification in ethics was the MA in Teaching Health Care Ethics run at the Institute of Education, University of London, during the 1990s. Interestingly, there still seems to be a need for such courses as evidenced by the recently introduced summer schools at the University of Surrey.

2   One former requirement of the NMC (2004) is that students emerging from pre-registration nursing programmes as registered nurses will have internalised the NMC code. In the revised Standards for Pre-registration Nursing Education (NMC 2010) the NMC has pulled back from insisting that students must internalise the code, but nevertheless indicates that by the time of completion of their course of study nursing students must practise in ways consistent with the code.

3   In the UK provision is made for individuals to begin a preparatory nursing programme at an age of no younger than 17 years and 6 months but in practice students are rarely younger than 18.

4   For a fuller discussion of this point but in relation to teaching see Carr 2003.

5   Milgram's experiment was conducted in the early 1960s in the attempt to understand why ordinary individuals would conform to orders requiring them to act in ways inconsistent with the usual norms of society.

6   For a more comprehensive account of stoic philosophy see Nussbaum (1994).

7   For an easily accessible account of the philosophy of Seneca see de Botton (2000).

8   See, for example, Griffin (1986, 1996), Parfitt (1984), Paul, Miller and Paul (1999).

9   In the UK the term registered nurse is protected in law and can be used only by someone whose name appears on the register of nursing practitioners held by the NMC.

10 For a detailed account of the 'state registration battle' see Abel-Smith (1960).

11 Baier is a little inconsistent at this point, for in a later part of her discussion she notes that infants do in fact demonstrate trust. I return to the issue of infant trust later in the same chapter.

12 I am grateful to Patricia White for this real life example.

13 The three texts I have in mind here are Cohen's *What's Wrong with Hospitals?* (1964); Martin's *Hospitals in Trouble* (1984) and Rob's *Sans Everything* (1967). Full references can be found in the reference list at the end of this book. There are, of course, other influential critical texts.

14 For a useful exploration of the relationship between personal and institutional trust see White 1996.

15 A lie is justified in this context in terms of what Potter understands as mainstream moral theory.

16 It should be noted that not all versions of virtue ethics accept this link between virtue and human flourishing. For a discussion of this point see, for example, Statman 1997.

17 By honest enquiry here I refer to enquiry as an attempt to find out about how things really are.

18 For a comprehensive account of the history of science illustrating the constant struggle for acceptance of ideas in spite what now seems compelling evidence see Gribbin (2002).

19 I am grateful to William Hare for suggesting this example as a possibility.

20 I am grateful to Terence McLaughlin for these suggested questions about which it might be inappropriate for nurses to be open-minded.

21 For example, the deliberate betrayal of the trust of children in the situation where a child needs but refuses to accept an important and necessary treatment or procedure has been reported as a widespread but apparently unproblematic 'fact' of children's nursing (Bircher 1999).

References

Abel-Smith, B. (1960) *A History of the Nursing Profession.* London: Heinemann.

ANA (American Nurses Association) (2001) *Code of Ethics for Nurses with Interpretive Statements.* Washington, DC: ANA.

Anderson, C. (2002) 'Workplace violence: are some nurses more vulnerable?' *Issues in Mental Health Nursing 23*, 4, 351–366.

Appleton, J.V. (1994) 'The concept of vulnerability in relation to child protection: health visitors' perceptions.' *Journal of Advanced Nursing 20*, 6, 1132–1140.

Aristotle (1953) *The Nichomachean Ethics.* Harmondsworth: Penguin.

Baier, A.C. (1985) *Postures of the Mind.* London: Methuen.

Baier, A.C. (1986) 'Trust and antitrust.' *Ethics 96*, 231–260.

Banks, S. (2001) *Ethics and Values in Social Work*, 2nd edn. Basingstoke: Palgrave.

Banks, S. and Gallagher, A. (2009) *Ethics in Professional Life: Virtues for Health and Social Care.* Basingstoke: Palgrave Macmillan.

Beauchamp, T.L. and Childress, J.F. (2008) *Principles of Biomedical Ethics*, 6th edn. Oxford: Oxford University Press.

Bircher, G. (1999) 'Paediatric nurses, children and the development of trust.' *Journal of Clinical Nursing 8*, 4, 451–458.

Bishop, A.H. and Scudder, J.R. (1991) *Nursing: The Practice of Caring.* New York: National League for Nursing Press.

Blum, L.A. (1980) *Friendship, Altruism and Morality.* London: Routledge and Kegan Paul.

Boston, P., Towers, A. and Barnard, D. (2001) 'Embracing vulnerability: risk and empathy in palliative care.' *Journal of Palliative Care 17*, 4, 248–253.

Bramall, S. (2000) 'Opening up open-mindedness.' *Educational Theory 50*, 2, 201–212.

Burnyeat, M.F. (1984) 'Aristotle: on Learning to Be Good.' In T. Honderich (ed.) *Philosophy through Its Past.* Harmondsworth: Penguin.

Callan, E. (1997) *Creating Citizens: Political Education and Liberal Democracy.* Oxford: Clarendon Press.

Carel, H. (2009) 'A reply to "Towards an understanding of nursing as a response to human vulnerability" by Derek Sellman: vulnerability and illness.' *Nursing Philosophy 10*, 3, 214–220.

Carlton, W. (1978) *In Our Professional Opinion… The Primacy of Clinical Judgment over Moral Choice.* Notre Dame: University of Notre Dame Press.

CARNA (College and Association of Registered Nurses of Alberta) (2010) *Guide to Registration Renewal 2011*, available at www.nurses.ab.ca/Carna/index. aspx?WebStructureID=4047 (accessed November 2010).

Carr, D. (1991) *Educating the Virtues: An Essay in the Philosophical Psychology of Moral Development and Education*. London: Routledge.

Carr, D. (2003) 'Moral educational implications of rival conceptions of education and the role of the teacher.' *Journal of Moral Education 32*, 3, 219–232.

Clarke, H.F. and Driever, M.J. (1983) 'Vulnerability: the Development of a Construct for Nursing.' In P.L. Chinn (ed.) *Advances in Nursing Theory Development*. Gaithersburg, MD: Aspen.

CNA (Canadian Nurses Association) (2008) *Code of Ethics for Registered Nurses*. Ottawa: CNA.

Cohen, G.L. (1964) *What's Wrong with Hospitals?* Harmondsworth: Penguin.

Daniel, L.E. (1998) 'Vulnerability as a key to authenticity.' *Image: Journal of Nursing Scholarship 30*, 2, 191.

Davis, G., August, S. and Salome, S. (1999) 'Nurses at risk a call to mobilize.' *American Journal of Nursing 99*, 5, 44–46.

De Botton, A. (2000) *The Consolations of Philosophy*. London: Hamish Hamilton.

De Raeve, L. (2002) 'The modification of emotional responses: a problem for trust in nurse–patient relationships?' *Nursing Ethics 9*, 5, 465–471.

DoH (Department of Health) (1999) *No Secrets. The Protection of Vulnerable Adults. Guidance on the Development and Implementation of Multi-agency Policy and Procedures*. London: DoH.

Dunne, J. (1999) 'Virtue, *Phronesis* and Learning.' In D. Carr and J. Steutel (eds) *Virtue Ethics and Moral Education*. London: Routledge.

Dunne, J. (2003) 'Arguing for teaching as a practice: a reply to Alasdair MacIntyre.' *Journal of Philosophy of Education 37*, 2, 353–369.

Durkheim, E. (1957) *Professional Ethics and Civic Morals*, trans. Cornelia Brookfield. London: Routledge.

Edwards, S.D. (2001) *Philosophy of Nursing. An Introduction*. Basingstoke: Palgrave.

Edwards, S.D. (2009) *Nursing Ethics A Principle-Based Approach*, 2nd edn. Basingstoke: Macmillan.

English National Board for Nursing, Midwifery and Health Visiting and Department of Health (2001) *Preparation of Mentors and Teachers. A New Framework of Guidance*. London: ENB and DoH.

Fawcett, J. (1983) 'Hallmarks of Success in Nursing Theory Development.' In P.L. Chinn (ed.) *Advances in Nursing Theory Development*. Gaithersburg, MD: Aspen.

Fukuyama, F. (1995) *Trust: The Social Virtues and the Creation of Prosperity*. London: Penguin.

Gardner, P. (1993) 'Should we teach children to be open-minded? Or is the pope open-minded about the existence of God?' *Journal of Philosophy of Education 27*, 1, 39–43.

Gilbert, T. (1998) 'Towards a politics of trust.' *Journal of Advanced Nursing 27*, 5, 1010–1016.

Gillon, R. (1985) *Philosophical Medical Ethics*. Chichester: John Wiley and Sons.

Gribbin, J. (2002) *Science A History*. Harmondsworth: Penguin.

Griffin, E. (2003) 'Oral chemotherapy: considerations for oncology nursing practice.' *Clinical Journal of Oncology Nursing* 7, 6, 25–29, 37–39.

Griffin, J. (1986) *Well-being: Its Meaning, Measurement and Moral Importance*. Oxford: Clarendon Press.

Griffin, J. (1996) *Value Judgement: Improving Our Ethical Beliefs*. Oxford: Clarendon Press.

Haack, S. (1998) *Manifesto of a Passionate Moderate*. Chicago: University of Chicago Press.

Hare, W. (1985) *In Defense of Open-mindedness*. Montreal: McGill-Queens University Press.

Hare, W. (1988) 'Open-mindedness in Elementary Education.' In W. Hare and J.P. Portelli (eds) *Philosophy of Education: Introductory Readings*. Calgary: Detselig Enterprises.

Hare, W. (2003) 'The ideal of open-mindedness and its place in education.' *Journal of Thought 38*, 2, 3–10.

Hare, W. and McLaughlin, T. (1994) 'Open-mindedness, commitment and Peter Gardner.' *Journal of Philosophy of Education 28*, 2, 239–244.

Harman, G. (1999) 'Moral philosophy meets social psychology virtue ethics and the fundamental attribution error.' *Proceedings of the Aristotelian Society 99*, 3, 315–331.

Hart, K. (1988) 'Kinship, Contract, and Trust: the Economic Organization of Migrants in an African City Slum.' In D. Gambetta (ed.) *Trust. Making and Breaking Cooperative Relations*. New York: Basil Blackwell.

Hek, G., Judd, M. and Moule, P. (2002) *Making Sense of Research. An Introduction for Health and Social Care Practitioners*, 2nd edn. London: Continuum.

Henderson, V. (1966) *The Nature of Nursing. A Definition and Its Implications for Practice, Research, and Education*. New York: Macmillan.

Holt, J. (2005) Personal email communication, 4 March.

Holt, J. and Long, T. (1999) 'Moral guidance, moral philosophy, and moral issues in practice.' *Nurse Education Today 19*, 3, 246–249.

Holton, R. (1994) 'Deciding to trust, coming to believe.' *Australian Journal of Philosophy 72*, 1, 63–75.

Hudson, T. (1998) *Key Stage 3 Classroom Science*. London: Letts Educational.

Humm, C. (2002) 'Self-preservation.' *Nursing Standard 16*, 26, 20.

Hursthouse, R. (1997) 'Virtue Theory and Abortion.' In D. Statman (ed.) *Virtue Ethics: A Critical Reader*. Edinburgh: Edinburgh University Press.

Hussey, T. (1990) 'Nursing ethics and project 2000.' *Journal of Advanced Nursing 15*, 12, 1377–1382.

Jackson, J. (2001) *Truth, Trust and Medicine*. London: Routledge.

Johns, J.L. (1996) 'A concept analysis of trust.' *Journal of Advanced Nursing 24*, 1, 76–83.

Kennedy, I. (2001) 'Summary of the final report of The Inquiry into the Management of Care of Children Receiving Complex Heart Surgery at the Bristol Royal Infirmary.' Available at www.bristol-inquiry.org.uk/final_report/index.htm (accessed November 2010).

Knight, K. (1998) 'Editor's Introduction.' In K. Knight (ed.) *The MacIntyre Reader.* Cambridge: Polity Press.

Koehn, D. (1994) *The Ground of Professional Ethics.* London: Routledge.

Kupperman, J.J. (2001) 'The indispensability of character.' *Philosophy 76*, 239–250.

Luhmann, N. (1988) 'Familiarity, Confidence, Trust: Problems and Alternatives.' In D. Gambetta (ed.) *Trust Making and Breaking Cooperative Relations.* New York: Basil Blackwell.

MacIntyre, A. (1975) 'How virtues become vices: values, medicine and social context.' In H. Engelhardt and S. Spicker (eds) *Evaluation and Explanation in the Biomedical Sciences.* Dordrecht: Reidel.

MacIntyre, A. (1985) *After Virtue: A Study in Moral Theory.* London: Duckworth.

MacIntyre, A. (1988) *Whose Justice? Which Rationality?* London: Duckworth.

MacIntyre, A. (1999) *Dependent Rational Animals. Why Human Beings Need the Virtues.* London: Duckworth.

MacIntyre, A. and Dunne, J. (2002) 'Alasdair MacIntyre on education: in dialogue with Joseph Dunne.' *Journal of Philosophy of Education 36*, 1, 1–19.

Malone, R. (2000) 'Dimensions of vulnerability in emergency nurses' narratives.' *Journal of Advanced Nursing 23*, 1, 1–11.

Martin, J.P. (ed.) (1984) *Hospitals in Trouble.* Oxford: Basil Blackwell.

Marton, F. and Saljo, R. (1976) 'On qualitative differences in learning. 1. Outcome and process.' *British Journal of Educational Psychology 46*, 4–11.

Maslow, A.H. (1968) *Toward a Psychology of Being.* New York: Van Nostrand Reinhold.

McLaughlin, T.H. (2003a) 'The Burdens and Dilemmas of Common Schooling.' In K. McDonough and W. Feinberg (eds) *Citizenship and Education in Liberal-Democratic Societies. Teaching for Cosmopolitan Values and Collective Identities.* Oxford: Oxford University Press.

McLaughlin, T.H. (2003b) 'Open-mindedness as an aim in moral education.' *Journal of Thought*, Summer, 21–32.

McLaughlin, T.H. (2005) 'Philosophy, Values and Schooling.' In W. Aiken and J. Haldane (eds) *Philosophy and its Public Role.* Exeter: Imprint Academic.

Meize-Grochowski, R. (1984) 'An analysis of the concept of trust.' *Journal of Advanced Nursing 9*, 6, 563–572.

Miller, D. (1994) 'Virtues, Practices and Justice.' In J. Horton and S. Mendus (eds) *After MacIntyre: Critical Perspectives on the Work of Alasdair MacIntyre.* Cambridge: Polity Press.

Munodawafa, D., Bower, D.A. and Webb, A.A. (1993) 'Perceived vulnerability to HIV/ AIDS in the US and Zimbabwe.' *International Nursing Review 40*, 1, 13–16, 24.

Nightingale, F. (1867) 'Extract from a letter to the editor of Macmillan's magazine April 1867', cited in M. Baly (1997) (ed.) *As Miss Nightingale Said…Florence Nightingale Through Her Sayings – A Victorian Perspective*, 2nd edn. London: Bailliere Tindall.

Nightingale, F. (1952) *Notes on Nursing.* London: Duckworth. (First published in 1859 as *Notes on Nursing: What it Is and What it is Not for the Labouring Classes.* London: Harrison).

NMC (Nursing and Midwifery Council) (undated) *Declaration of Good Health and Good Character in Support of an Application for Admission to a Part of the NMC's Professional Register.* London: NMC.

NMC (2002a) 'Accountability never sleeps.' *NMC News 3,* 9.

NMC (2002b) *Practitioner–Client Relationships and the Prevention of Abuse.* London: NMC.

NMC (2004) *Standards of Proficiency for Pre-registration Nursing Education.* London: NMC.

NMC (2008a) 'Good health and good character: guidance for educational institutions.' Available at www.nmc-uk.org/Educators/Good-health-and-good-character/ (accessed November 2010).

NMC (2008b) *The Code: Standards of Conduct, Performance and Ethics for Nurses and Midwives.* London: NMC.

NMC (2010) 'Standards for pre-registration nursing education.' Available at http://standards.nmc-uk.org/Pages/Downloads.aspx (accessed November 2010).

Noddings, N. and Slote, M. (2003) 'Changing Notions of the Moral and of Moral Education.' In N. Blake, P. Smeyers, R. Smith and P. Standish (eds) *The Blackwell Guide to The Philosophy of Education.* Malden, MA: Blackwell Publishing.

Nussbaum, M.C. (1994) *The Therapy of Desire. Theory and Practice in Hellenistic Ethics.* Princeton, NJ: Princeton University Press.

O'Hear, A. (1998) 'Moral Education.' In P.H. Hirst and P. White (eds) *Philosophy of Education. Major Themes in the Analytic Tradition. Volume IV. Problems of Educational Content and Practices.* London: Routledge.

O'Neill, O. (2002) *Autonomy and Trust in Bioethics.* Cambridge: Cambridge University Press.

Parfit, D. (1984) *Reasons and Persons.* Oxford: Clarendon Press.

Parish, C. (2000) 'Too close for comfort.' *Nursing Standard 15,* 2, 12–13.

Paul, E.F., Miller, F.D. and Paul, F. (eds) (1999) *Human Flourishing.* Social Philosophy and Policy 16, 1. New York: Cambridge University Press.

Payne, N. (2001) 'Occupational stressors and coping as determinants of burnout in female hospice nurses.' *Journal of Advanced Nursing 33,* 3, 396–405.

Potter, N.N. (2002) *How Can I Be Trusted? A Virtue Theory of Trustworthiness.* Lanham, MD: Rowan and Littlefield.

Quinn, C.A. (1990) 'A conceptual approach to the identification of essential ethics content for the undergraduate nursing curriculum.' *Journal of Advanced Nursing 15,* 6, 726–731.

RCN (Royal College of Nursing) (2002) *RCN Code of Practice for Patient Handling,* 2nd edn. London: RCN.

RCN (2003) *Defining Nursing.* London: RCN. Available at www.rcn.org.uk/__data/assets/pdf_file/0008/78569/001998.pdf (accessed November 2010).

Rob, B. (1967) *Sans Everything. A Case to Answer.* London: Nelson.

Royal College of Nursing Research Society (2003) 'Nurses and research ethics.' *Nurse Researcher 11,* 1, 7–21.

Rogers, R., Savage, J. and Cowell, R. (1998) 'Reducing the risk of hepatitis to staff.' *Professional Nurse 14*, 3, 193–6.

Redding, G.S. (1990) *The Spirit of Chinese Capitalism.* Berlin: DeGruyter.

Ryle, G. (1972) 'Can Virtue Be Taught?' In R.F. Dearden, P.H. Hirst and R.S. Peters (eds) *Education and The Development of Reason.* London: Routledge and Kegan Paul.

Scott, P.A. (1995) 'Aristotle, nursing and health care ethics.' *Nursing Ethics 2*, 4, 279–285.

Seedhouse, D. (2000) *Practical Nursing Philosophy: The Universal Ethical Code.* Chichester: John Wiley and Sons.

Seedhouse, D. (2009) *Ethics the Heart of Healthcare*, 3rd edn. Chichester: Wiley-Blackwell.

Seligman, A.B. (1997) *The Problem of Trust.* Princeton, NJ: Princeton University Press.

Sellman, D. (1996) 'Why teach ethics to nurses?' *Nurse Education Today 16*, 1, 44–48.

Sellman, D. (1997) 'The virtues in the moral education of nurses: Florence Nightingale revisited.' *Nursing Ethics 4*, 1, 3–11.

Sellman, D. (2000) 'Alasdair MacIntyre and the professional practice of nursing.' *Nursing Philosophy 1*, 1, 26–33.

Sellman, D. (2007) 'On being of good character: nurse education and the assessment of good character.' *Nurse Education Today 27*, 762–767.

Sellman, D. (2008) 'Teaching Ethics to Nurses in Higher Education: Just Another Subject or an Exercise in Moral Education.' In S. Robinson and J. Strain (eds) *Ethics for Living and Working.* Leicester: Troubador.

Sellman, D. (2009) 'Practical wisdom in health and social care: teaching for *professional phronesis*.' *Learning in Health and Social Care 8*, 2, 84–91.

Sellman, D. (2010) 'Values and Adult General Nursing.' In S. Pattison, B. Hannigan, R. Pill and H. Thomas (eds) *Emerging Values in Health Care: The Challenge for Professionals.* London: Jessica Kingsley Publishers.

Smith, C. (2001) 'Trust and confidence: possibilities for social work in "high modernity".' *British Journal of Social Work 31*, 287–305.

Sockett, H. (1993) *The Moral Base for Teacher Professionalism.* NewYork: Teachers College Press.

Statman, D. (1997) 'Introduction to Virtue Ethics.' In D. Statman (ed.) *Virtue Ethics: A Critical Reader.* Edinburgh: Edinburgh University Press.

Steutel, J. and Carr, D. (1999) 'Virtue Ethics and the Virtue Approach to Moral Education.' In D. Carr and J. Steutel (eds) *Virtue Ethics and Moral Education.* Routledge: London.

Steutel, J. and Spiecker, B. (2005) 'Cultivating sentimental dispositions through Aristotelian habituation.' *Journal of Philosophy of Education 38*, 4, 531–549.

Thompson, I.E., Melia, K.M. and Boyd, K.M. (2000) *Nursing Ethics*, 4th edn. Edinburgh: Churchill Livingstone.

Thorne, S.E. and Robinson, C.A. (1988) 'Reciprocal trust in heath care relationships.' *Journal of Advanced Nursing 13*, 6, 782–789.

Tschudin, V. (1992) *Ethics in Nursing: The Caring Relationship*, 2nd edn. Oxford: Butterworth Heinemann.

Turner, B.S. (1992) 'Preface to the Second Edition.' In E. Durkheim *Professional Ethics and Civic Morals*, trans. Cornelia Brookfield, 2nd edn. London: Routledge.

UKCC (United Kingdom Central Council for Nurses, Midwifery and Health Visiting) (1983) *Code of Professional Conduct for the Nurse Midwife and Health Visitor.* London: UKCC.

UKCC (1986) *Project 2000: A New Preparation for Nursing, Midwifery and Health Visiting.* London: UKCC.

Wainwright, P. (1997) 'The practice of nursing: an investigation of professional nursing from the perspective of the virtues ethics of Alasdair MacIntyre.' Unpublished PhD thesis, University of Wales, Swansea.

Wainwright, P. (2000) 'Critical response to Sellman's paper.' *Nursing Philosophy 1*, 1, 34–35.

Walsh, M. and Ford, P. (1989) *Nursing Rituals. Research and Rational Actions.* Oxford: Butterworth Heinemann.

West, M.M. (2002) 'Early risk indicators of substance abuse among nurses.' *Journal of Nursing Scholarship 34*, 2, 187–193.

White, P. (1996) *Civic Virtues and Public Schooling.* New York: Teachers College Press.

Williams, B. (2002) *Truth and Truthfulness.* Princeton, NJ: Princeton University Press.

Wilson, J., Williams, N. and Sugarman, B. (1967) *Introduction to Moral Education.* Harmondsworth: Penguin.

Winstanley, S. and Whittington, R. (2004) 'Aggression towards health care staff in a UK general hospital: variation among professions and departments.' *Journal of Clinical Nursing 13*, 1, 3–10.

Wolpert, L. (1992) *The Unnatural Nature of Science.* London: Faber and Faber.

Woods, M. (2005) 'Nursing ethics education: are we really delivering the good(s)?' *Nursing Ethics 12*, 1, 5–18.

Woogara, J. (2005) 'International Centre for Nursing Ethics summer school: teaching ethics to healthcare students, 21–23 July 2004, European Institute of Health and Medical Sciences, University of Surrey, Guildford, UK.' *Nursing Ethics 12*, 1, 108–109.

Wray, H. (1962) *Ethics for Nurses.* London: Macmillan Journals Limited.

Subject Index

justification-oriented ethics 146

Kantian morality 115
kinship, trust 129
'know when' 38
knowledge
    propositional and
        practical 38, 189
    and trust 139
Kohlbergian approach 32

late adolescence, moral
    education 35
learning, deep 90
lecturers 193, 195–6
legitimacy, of evidence 175
liberal democracy 34
liberalism 162
luck 53, 54

Martin Chuzzlewit 37
Maslow's hierarchy 51
mean, aiming for 119, 161
medical ethics 30
medical information
    control of 123
    withholding 123
    see also information
medicine
    conservatism 123
    trust in 122–3
mentors 193, 195
misplaced trust 118
modernity, fragmentation of
    46, 47–8, 83, 178
moral action 183
moral agency 183–5, 198,
    202
moral apartheid 89, 91
moral behaviour, basis for
    148
moral content 20–1
moral education 19, 27,
    34–6, 39
    general and nursing 194
    nature of 179–80
    nursing education as
        179–80

or moral training 182–5,
    202
purpose of 181
role of institutions
    205–6
understanding 184–5
moral guidance 31–3
moral practice, teaching
    for 191
moral theory, Potter's
    critique 146–8
moral training 180
    or moral education 182–
    5, 202
more-than-ordinarily
    vulnerable persons 18,
    24, 49, 51, 59–61
    abuse of trust of 134
    human flourishing 77,
        88–90, 91, 100
    and morality of nursing
        177
    nurses as witnesses of
        73–5
    patients as 67–8, 203
    protection 69, 70
    trust 120–1
    see also vulnerability
motivation 55–6, 101–2
mutuality 143–4

Nichomachean Ethics 36, 167,
    188
Nightingale, Florence 28,
    36, 95
nomenclature 21–2
nonmutuality 143–4
nurse teachers 29, 192–5
nurses
    occupational hazards 71,
        72–3
    as possible abusers
        69–70
    public trust 69
    vulnerability of 71–5
    as witnesses of
        vulnerability 73–5
nursing
    as art 95

complexity of 76–7
defining 93–6
as extraordinary 148
as inherently moral 177
as MacIntyrean practice
    93–104, 177, 178,
    203
as practical activity 38
as practice 20
as a practice 100–4
problem of definition 20,
    22–3, 24
range and scope 94–5
risk and vulnerability 63
as science 22–3, 24,
    95–100, 102
theories of 95–6
trust in 130–1
virtues 179
Nursing and Midwifery
    Council (NMC) 46,
    69–70
character requirements
    19
declaration of good
    character 204–5
nursing codes 23, 76,
    105–6, 205
character development
    27
trustworthiness 46, 108
UKCC 29
nursing education
    approaches to 25
    intellectual virtue 190–1
    moral education 179–80
    moral education or moral
        training 182–5
    moral nature 202
    moral practice 191
    nature of moral education
        180–1
    open-mindedness 200–2
    overview 177–9
    for professional virtue
        47–8
    teaching for good will
        186–7

Author Index

American Nurses
   Association (ANA) 76,
   108
Anderson, C. 71
Appleton, J.V. 61
Aristotle 36, 38, 167
August, S. 71

Baier, A.C. 30, 108, 109, 110,
   111, 112, 113, 114–17,
   120–1, 125, 129, 130,
   133, 134, 138
Banks, S. 108, 126–8
Barnard, D. 73
Beauchamp, T.L. 29, 146
Bishop, A.H. 100–1, 102
Blum, L.A. 145
Boston, P. 73
Bower, D.A. 71
Boyd, K.M. 29
Bramall, S. 164–5
Burnyeat, M.F. 36, 187

Callan, E. 35
Canadian Nurses
   Association (CNA) 76,
   106, 108
Carel, H. 60, 73, 75
Carlton, W. 122
Carr, D. 34, 178, 180, 181
Childress, J.F. 29, 146
Clarke, H.F. 62–7
College and Association of
   Registered Nurses of
   Alberta (CARNA) 19
Cowell, R. 71

Daniel, L.E. 73–4
Davis, G. 71
De Raeve, L. 126–7
Department of Health (DH)
   69, 193
Dickens, Charles 37
Dreiver, M.J. 62–7
Dunne, J. 20, 84–5, 187,
   190

Edwards, S.D. 29, 43, 97,
   98, 101, 102
English National Board for
   Nursing, Midwifery
   and Health Visiting
   (ENB) 193

Fawcett, J. 62
Ford, P. 166
Fukuyama, F. 129

Gallagher, A. 108
Gardner, P. 153–6, 158,
   161, 163
Gilbert, T. 125–6, 133
Gillon, R. 29
Griffin, J. 71

Haack, S. 171
Hare, W. 153, 156, 158,
   163
Harman, G. 40–4
Hart, K. 113–14
Hek, G. 175, 197
Henderson, V. 94, 95
Holt, J. 29, 31–3

Holton, R. 112, 114–15,
   116–17
Hudson, T. 97
Humm, C. 71
Hursthouse, R. 40
Hussey, T. 43

Jackson, J. 147
Johns, J.L. 133
Judd, M. 175

Kennedy, I. 124–5
Knight, K. 80
Koehn, D. 35
Kupperman, J.J. 42–3

Long, T. 29, 31–3
Luhmann, N. 117

MacIntyre, A. 19–20,
   24, 46, 77, 78–86,
   87–93, 101, 102–3,
   104–7, 126–8, 133,
   142, 150, 152, 165,
   171, 173, 177, 178,
   188, 195, 203, 206
McLaughlin, T.H. 18, 34,
   38, 156, 163, 170,
   200
Malone, R. 73
Marton, F. 90
Maslow, A. 51
Meize-Grochowski, R. 133
Melia, K.M. 29
Milgram, S. 41
Miller, D. 82–4